TOTAL HEALTH

How to Unlock Your Body's Natural Ability to Burn Fat, Stay Healthy &

BOOST YOUR ENERGY

Dr. Douglas J. Markham

 Total Health Care Partners, Inc., Westlake Village, California

First Edition

Library of Congress Catalog Card Number 00-192101
Publisher's Cataloging-in-Publication
(Provided by Quality Books, Inc.)

Markham, Douglas J.
   Total Health Beyond the Zone: how to unlock your body's natural
ability to burn fat, stay healthy & boost your energy /
by Douglas J. Markham.
   -- 1st ed.
   p. cm.
   Includes bibliographical references and index.

   ISBN: 0-9701710-3-X

   1. Health. 2. Nutrition. 3. Physical fitness. I. Title.

RA76.M37 2001   613.7
                    QBI00-746

Dedication

To my wife and best friend, Andrea R. Gasporra, D.D.S. for her never-ending love, patience and understanding.

To Bruce and Helen Timm, the neighbors whose love and generosity made all the difference in a young boy's life.

For my grandmother, Mary Markham, who was born on a Wisconsin farm in 1898 and who lived to age 94. Her stories, guidance, and family values continue to influence and inspire me.

Acknowledgements

I want to express my gratitude to the many people who made this book possible, starting with my patients and friends, who urged me to share the Total Health eating and wellness program with the rest of the world. This book would not exist without their unwavering support. In particular, I'd like to thank the people whose time, talent and dedication helped shape and polish the pages that follow.

Paul C. Reisser, M.D., family practice, and former Chief of Staff, Los Robles Regional Medical Center, for his continuing professional support, sound medical advice and insightful review of this manuscript.

Frank M. Dawson, M.D., family practice, for somehow finding time between his family, practice and his tireless work with the Conejo Free Clinic to write the foreword.

Thanks also to Stephen G. Axelrode, D.O., family practice, Chief of Primary Care, Los Robles Regional Medical Center, and Robert J. Wallace, M.D., Obstetrics/ Gynecology, Peer Review Committee Chair, Los Robles Regional Medical Center, for their patient referrals and professional feedback.

I am also grateful to Shirley O'Donnell, R.N., Amgen occupational health services, for her helpful manuscript suggestions; to Laurel Burns, R.N., M.S., manager of health services for Procter and Gamble, for supporting Total Health as an employee benefit and internet-based corporate wellness program; and to Valerie McCormick, vice president of operations, Sage Publications, for her early support of this book and the Total Health program.

Thanks to Robert Shaw, chief executive officer, Los Robles Regional Medical Center, for helping me introduce the Total Health program to the medical community and to his wife, Lisa, who has championed Total Health's benefits to youth through local Parent Teacher's Associations.

Special thanks to Faye Mallinger, M.S., MFT, for her insight and contributions to the chapter on mental health; to Klay Hall, director of animation, Fox Television Network, for his friendship, enthusiasm, and encouragement; and to Marc Colen, intellectual property attorney, for his direction, guidance, and friendship throughout this project.

Ethan Blumen of Clarity Communications, for his friendship, editorial direction and boundless enthusiasm for this program and its ability to change people's lives.

Praise is also due Kevin Plambeck, director of marketing, Gateway Arts, for his good humor, good taste and financial acumen while marshalling this book through production, and for introducing me to Stephanie Spruch, whose design and illustrations grace these pages.

TOTAL HEALTH

How to Unlock Your Body's Natural Ability to Burn Fat, Stay Healthy &
BOOST YOUR ENERGY

Table of Contents

	Foreword	**9**
	Introduction	**11**
1	What You Will Learn	**17**
2	Food Is a Drug: The Hormonal Connection	**21**
3	Eating Your Way to Health	**25**
4	Exercise: How to Get Started and Why	**61**
5	Mental Health: Helpful Hints for Happiness	**77**
6	Total Health Success Stories	**85**
	Appendix I: Commit to Health and Happiness!	**101**
	Appendix II: Total Health Before and After Photos	**103**
	Bibliography	**111**
	Index	**113**

Foreword

As a medical doctor specializing in family practice, I'm always looking for simple and effective ways to help my patients live healthier lives.

For years, I've been referring my patients to Dr. Markham for his chiropractic expertise and manipulation skills. Now I also refer patients specifically for his nutritional counseling.

When Dr. Markham first told me about the results his patients were achieving with his protein-rich, favorable-carbohydrate eating program, I was cautiously optimistic. I've been practicing family medicine since 1978. Over the years, I've seen how obesity often leads to high blood pressure, diabetes and other serious health risks. I've seen patients struggle to lose excess weight. I've also seen a lot of diets fail.

Dr. Markham's Total Health program works because it is not a diet. It's a sensible, sustainable way of eating based on proven nutritional principles, practical real-world experience and results. After losing weight by following the Total Health program, some of my patients have lowered their blood pressure and cholesterol levels significantly. As a result, they no longer need to take high blood pressure or cholesterol medicine.

If you're looking for a safe, dependable way to lose ten or twenty pounds, the Total Health program can help you change your waist size. And if you are obese or you suffer from high blood pressure, high cholesterol or type II diabetes, the information in this book can change your life.

Here's to your health!

Frank Dawson, M.D.
Thousand Oaks, California
November 2000

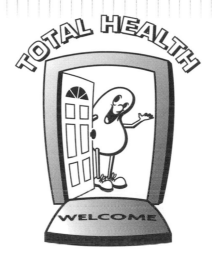

C ongratulations! If you are reading these words, you've taken a giant step towards taking control of your health and improving the quality and length of your life. This is especially true if you are overweight.

If you have been trying to lose 10-15-25- even 40 or more pounds, you're not alone. More than one in three Americans is clinically obese. In June 1998, the government adopted a new, much more strict, clinical criteria to determine who is overweight and who is obese. As a result, another 25 million Americans became "fat" overnight.

Although the government's new obesity guidelines are based on a controversial formula, what's really important is the reason behind the new criteria. And the reason is simple...

Obesity is a serious, serious health risk. Obesity is a major risk factor for heart disease and heart attack. It's also a known risk factor for chronic diseases such as diabetes, high blood pressure, stroke, breast and colon cancer.

How many times have you dropped and gained the same 15, 20 or 50 pounds?

The harsh reality is that the extra weight you carry can kill you.

"Obesity contributes to more than 300,000 excess deaths each year," says George Blackburn, president of the American Society of Clinical Nutrition. "Next to smoking, obesity is the second-leading cause of preventable death in the United States."

That's worth repeating: Next to smoking, obesity is the second-leading cause of preventable death in the United States!

But it's not really news that being overweight or obese is bad for you, is it? Losing weight is something most of us have tried to do — usually more than once. You drop the weight — and after a while — you put it right back on.

How many times have you dropped and gained the same 15, 25 or 50 pounds?

It's frustrating.
It's embarrassing.
And it can be expensive.

How many books have you bought? How many weight loss programs have you paid for? The weight loss industry in America is a $33 billion industry. That's billion with a "B." How much of that came out of your pocket? Probably too much.

If you're a veteran of the weight-loss wars, someone who's read the books, attended the meetings, counted the calories and fiddled with fads and magic pills, the question you must answer is WHY? Why do you keep trying to lose weight? Why not abandon all hope and dive head-first into a crate of chocolate donuts?

The answer to that question probably goes deeper than wanting to fit into nicer clothes. Or trying to get a handle on runaway blood pressure. It also runs deeper than wanting to stay alive for the loved ones in your life.

Ultimately, the reason you keep trying is that you believe you have the absolute right to be healthy and happy. This belief — that we have an absolute right to be healthy and happy — is also a driving force in my life. It's the reason I became a doctor. And it was my personal and professional pursuit of this idea that led me to introduce my patients to the material you are about to read.

> **... you have the absolute right to be healthy and happy.**

Several years ago, I had the opportunity to work in a medical office with doctors who specialized in family practice. We referred a number of patients to each other. Many of our "shared" patients suffered from problems caused by obesity, such as high blood pressure, high cholesterol, and diabetes — conditions that these patients preferred to address through lifestyle changes in diet and exercise rather than medication.

So the M.D.s recommended a low-fat, high-carbohydrate diet and exercise program — an approach that was popular at the time. But there was a problem.

It wasn't working.

Even though our patients were following the classic low-fat, high-carbohydrate nutritional guidelines promoted by the healthcare community, they were not losing much weight. They were not regulating their blood sugar levels. They were not lowering cholesterol or reducing their blood pressure.

The dramatic results I began to see in my patients were nothing short of life changing .

At the same time, I began to have some health problems of my own. Namely, I couldn't keep my energy levels up. I've always been a very active person. In high school, I was an All-American wrestler. And as a doctor, one of my passions was cross-training for triathlons. So I was riding my bike, swimming and running. I was also training a couple mornings a week in an obscure form of Brazilian Jujitsu. I was juicing. I was taking my supplements.

And I was on my high-carb, low-fat diet. When it came to training and nutrition, I was doing everything right. I figured I should be a superhuman. Instead I was exhausted.

I'd have my high-carb meal — the pasta with the low-fat red sauce — and some veggies, and about half an hour later, I felt like I needed to take a nap. I knew something was wrong. I even had my blood tested for anemia.

About the same time, I became aware of nutritional principles popularized by best-selling books such as *Enter The Zone* by Barry Sears, Ph.D., and *Protein Power* by Micheal Eades, M.D. and Mary Eades, M.D. According to these books, you could increase your energy levels by regulating your blood sugars.

The key was to eat protein-rich, favorable-carbohydrate meals. Not eliminating all carbohydrates, just increasing the protein and easing off the unfavorable forms of carbohydrates.

So I decided to give "The Zone" a try. For one thing, the physiology behind this way of eating made sense. For another, this was a balanced approach to eating — not some extreme alternative like diet pills or liquid meals.

The results were fantastic. Within about two weeks my energy levels soared. I also lost about five pounds around the middle. Remember, all I wanted was more energy. The weight loss was a bonus! Most of all, I was excited about the prospect of sharing this information with my patients.

But unfortunately, I couldn't tell my patients to go out and buy these books because they were too technical for most people to understand. So I did more research, and used my personal experience to make this exciting information accessible and easy to use in the real world.

The dramatic results I began to see in my patients were nothing short of life changing. Patients who were obese have lost the weight. In many cases, their M.D.s have taken them off their high blood pressure medications, their diabetes medications and their cholesterol medications. And the weight has stayed off. Total Health is not some fad diet. It's a way of eating that will work for the rest of your life.

And by the way, it's increasingly clear what does not work. The old way of eating. I'm talking about the classic high-carb, low-fat diet that leading nutritionists, government experts and diet gurus have been drilling into our heads for more than 15 years.

How do we know it doesn't work? Well, for the last 15 years, membership at health clubs has skyrocketed. The fitness equipment industry is booming. And as a nation, we're about 32 percent fatter today than we were 15 years ago.

If you like to go by results — and I certainly do — that means the nutritional information we've been getting isn't working.

The nutritional principles behind Total Health do work. It's worked for me, it's worked for hundreds of my patients. And it can work for you.

1 What You Will Learn

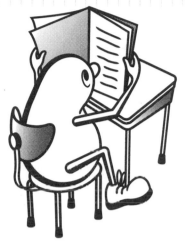

One of the reasons that the Total Health program works is that it is a simple, common sense way to burn fat, increase your energy levels and boost your immune system through proper diet and exercise.

Much of what has been written about the nutritional principles behind Total Health is either too technical or too full of hype. That's why my patients kept after me to write a no nonsense book about how to make this program work.

Hence, *Total Health: How to Unlock Your Body's Natural Ability to Burn Fat, Stay Healthy & Boost Your Energy.*

On the following pages, you'll find a straightforward explanation of the science behind Total Health. Use this book to review how the program works and to inspire your own success.

The material is organized into the following chapters:

• **Food Is a Drug: The Hormonal Connection.** The kind of food you eat has a tremendous affect on your body, your energy level, your mental alertness and the quality of your life. Like a drug, the food you eat causes powerful biochemical reactions in your body. You'll learn more about those reactions in a moment, but here's the bottom line:

> The kind of food you eat and the amount of food you eat and when you eat it tells your body whether to burn fat or store fat.

• **Eating Your Way to Health.** You'll learn how the right balance of carbohydrates, protein and fat can help you boost your energy, lose weight and stay healthy. You're also going to learn about the kind of micronutrients to look for in vitamin and mineral supplements.

• **Exercise: How to Get Started and Why.** You'll learn how a combination of aerobic, resistance and passive exercise will make your body stronger and keep it working longer. I'll also give you insider tips on choosing a health club and working with a personal trainer.

• **Mental Health: Helpful Hints for Happiness.** This chapter offers a few thoughts about the importance of exercising that big muscle between your ears. Remember, you have the absolute right to be healthy and HAPPY. One of the keys to Total Health is that your mental health is just as important as your physical health.

• **Total Health Success Stories.** Need some inspiration or motivation? Skeptical? The Total Health program is working for everyday people every day! In this chapter, you'll read the stories of six patients who have changed their lives using the Total Health program.

• **Appendix I: Commit to Health and Happiness.**

• **Appendix II: Total Health Before and After Photos.**

One Final Note: The Total Health program is subject to modifications based on new developments in nutrition and medicine. This book contains information that is current at the time of printing. For the latest updates and information, visit out Web site: **www.totalhealthdoc.com**

2 Food Is a Drug: The Hormonal Connection

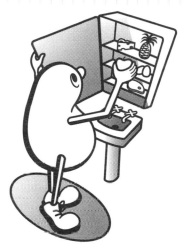

Being aware of the connection between your health and what you eat is the first step to living in total health. So, repeat these words out loud: "Food is a drug."

Don't believe me? After you've read this chapter, not only will you agree with me, you'll also understand why food is among the most dangerous "over-the-counter" drugs available.

How is food like a drug? First, like a drug, food can be addictive. Second, like a drug, food causes strong biochemical reactions in your body. And finally, like a drug, food can be used or abused. Take an over-the-counter cough syrup, for example. Use it in the proper dosage for the right reason, and you can tame your cough. But start drinking the stuff like water…and a cough is the least of your problems.

We all know how easy it is to abuse food. For many people, there are strong psychological forces behind their eating behavior. Those issues need to be worked out with professional help. But, the impulse to eat certain kinds of foods is not all in your head. When you get the craving for those M&Ms in the bottom right desk drawer, there's some serious biochemistry at work, too.

Blame your hormones.

The Hormonal Connection

Hormones are chemicals manufactured by special glands in your body and released into your bloodstream. Your blood transports hormones to different parts of your body, where hormones influence the way certain organs and tissues work.

> **. . . the kind of food you eat, and how much you eat triggers the release of two powerful hormones, insulin and glucagon.**

Because hormones control and influence so many vital processes — such as growth, sexual drive and aging to name just a few — hormone research is one of the most exciting fields of medical science. Among the scientific knowledge to emerge from these studies is the strong connection between food and hormones. Specifically, the kind of food you eat — and how much you eat — triggers the release of two powerful hormones, insulin and glucagon.

What, you may ask, is so important about insulin and glucagon? The answer is simple: Insulin tells your body to store fat. Glucagon tells your body to burn fat.

If you are overweight or you always feel tired after meals, chances are that you are eating foods or an amount of food that causes your body to produce too much insulin.

This is not good.

The Dangers of Excess Insulin

When you eat foods that produce too much insulin, not only are you telling your body to store fat, all that excess insulin boosts production of triglycerides or blood fats. And what does blood fat do to your arteries? It clogs them, which makes you a prime candidate for a stroke or heart attack.

Excess insulin also stimulates the liver to produce cholesterol. This is why your cholesterol levels can still be high *even if you cut all the fats out of your diet.* The amount of fat you eat does not influence your blood cholesterol levels that much. The real culprit is excess insulin, which also contributes to high blood pressure.

I've saved the worst for last. When your body produces excess insulin on a regular basis, you're likely to develop insulin resistance. This is a vicious cycle where the body becomes less sensitive to insulin and compensates by secreting more and more of the stuff. The result: You store more and more fat and gain more and more weight. After a while, your pancreas, which produces insulin, cannot satisfy the demand. This is a precursor to acquiring a deadly disease called adult onset diabetes.

Adult onset diabetes, also known as type II diabetes, affects more than eight million Americans. It is a devastating disease characterized by loss of energy and weight gain. People afflicted with diabetes suffer blindness, heart disease, kidney failure and circulatory problems that often lead to the amputation of fingers and toes. Diabetes is also a well known cause of male impotency.

Scared? You should be. It's estimated that there are another eight million Americans who suffer from some form of diabetes and don't even know it!

The Good News

Now, take a deep breath. There is a proven way to get your body to reduce the amount of fat-storing insulin and promote the release of fat-burning glucagon. And you don't need expensive prescription medicines or pre-packaged meals. The secret, as you'll learn in the next chapter, is to eat the right combination of everyday foods, in the right amount, at the right time.

3 Eating Your Way to Health

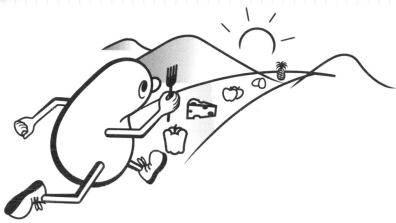

To understand why Total Health works to burn fat, boost your energy and keep you healthy, we need to take a quick look at how your body converts food into energy and fat.

All food is composed of macronutrients (carbohydrates, proteins and fat), micronutrients (vitamins, minerals and trace elements) and water. Macronutrients provide energy as food is digested through a series of complex chemical reactions. Micronutrients help the body process and dispose of the macronutrients more efficiently.

Part 1 of this chapter deals with the heart of the Total Health program — eating a proper balance of carbohydrates, proteins and fats. In Part 2, we'll sort through the hype about vitamin and mineral supplements. You'll also learn how much water and fiber your body really needs.

Part 1: Macronutrients

Carbohydrates are found in high amounts in foods such as bread, pasta, fruits, juices, vegetables and sweets. When you eat carbohydrate-rich foods, your body converts them into glucose, also known as blood sugar.

Protein is food such as beef, poultry, fish, pork, soy and dairy products such as eggs and cheese. Protein is made of amino acids, which your body uses to repair itself. Nine of these amino acids, known as the essential amino acids, cannot be synthesized by your body and must be supplied by a high-quality protein diet.

Fats are foods such as butter, oil, and the fat on red meat. The important thing to know about fat is that it's not all bad. In fact, you need the *right kind* of fat in your diet in the *right* amount to burn body fat and produce hormones essential to good health.

The Hormonal Response to Food

In the introduction of this book, I declared that the classic high-carbohydrate, low-fat diet does not work. One reason is that most people think that all you have to do to lose weight is cut out all the dietary fat. Well, here's another bit of nutritional heresy: Fat does not make you fat!

Fat does not make you fat.

That's right! Contrary to what nutritionists and the media have been spouting for decades, eating fat is not the reason so many Americans are overweight. The real culprit is the high carbohydrate content of our diet.

> This high-carb fat connection isn't news to at least one segment of the food industry — livestock farmers. I grew up in Wisconsin, and as any pig or cattle farmer will tell you, you don't use fat to plump up the herd. You use low-fat grain!

The reason excess carbohydrate consumption leads to obesity has to do with your body's hormonal response to food. Here's what happens when you eat a meal that is loaded with carbohydrates.

When you eat a high-carbohydrate meal, like pasta or French toast or half a box of Ding Dongs, those carbs are rapidly converted into glucose or blood sugar. As a result, your blood sugar levels surge. At first, this makes your brain very happy. The brain is a glucose hog and consumes about two-thirds of the glucose in your body for energy.

The spike in blood sugar also triggers your pancreas to secrete insulin. Remember, insulin's job is to reduce the amount of glucose in the bloodstream. It does this by storing excess glucose. First, a small amount is stored in your liver and muscles. The rest of the excess glucose is stored as body fat.

But it's not over yet. As I said, the brain craves glucose. And when insulin does its job to reduce excess glucose, there isn't enough glucose left for the brain to convert into energy. This is why you start to nod off after a big carb-heavy meal.

So, the brain sends a message: consume more carbohydrates! That's when you reach for your mid-morning or mid-afternoon stash of M&Ms. That's how you end up taking a ride on the blood sugar roller coaster, cycling dramatically from high to low energy. And that's how all those excess carbs become excess pounds. It's a vicious cycle that leads to obesity, insulin resistance, hypoglycemia and worse.

> The secret to breaking this cycle and taking control of your health is simple: Increase the amount of protein you eat and decrease the amount of carbohydrates.

Eating the right amount of protein stimulates the release of glucagon, a hormone that helps stabilize your energy levels by mobilizing the release of the sugars stored in your liver to satisfy your brain's need for glucose. (Thus, curbing and eventually ending your carbohydrate cravings.) Another bonus: Glucagon also helps your body burn stored body fat!

So instead of eating French toast for breakfast, have an omelette with fresh fruit. Instead of pasta for lunch, eat chicken, beef or fish with vegetables.

Now don't get me wrong. I'm not saying that all carbohydrates are bad for you. Carbohydrates are an essential part of healthy nutrition, as long as you eat the right amount and the right kind.

What makes one form of carbohydrate better than another? The answer is a carbohydrate's glycemic index — the rate at which a carbohydrate is converted into glucose, or sugar, in the bloodstream. *High-glycemic carbs* convert into sugar rapidly, causing an increased insulin response. *Low-glycemic carbs* convert into sugar at a slower rate, resulting in a reduced insulin response.

Carbohydrates are an essential part of healthy nutrition, as long as you eat the right amount and the right kind.

"Good" carbohydrates are low-glycemic carbohdrates. "Bad" carbohydrates are high-glycemic carbohydrates. If you want to live in total health, it is essential that you choose to eat good carbohydrates over bad carbohydrates whenever possible.

Virtually all fiber-rich fruits and vegetables are low-glycemic except for carrots, corn, dried fruits and bananas. Those are the fruits and vegetables you want to try and reduce in your diet. You also want to limit other carbohydrates that convert rapidly into sugar, such as bread, pasta, rice and potatoes. These foods are not entirely forbidden, but the less of them you eat, the better you'll feel.

Note: All patients receive a comprehensive list of favorable carbohydrates with their customized Total Health menu choices. These menus are also available at our Web site: **www.totalhealthdoc.com**

Okay, we've discussed carbohydrates and protein and how the hormonal responses these nutrients trigger influence your energy levels and whether your body stores fat or burns fat. Now, let's take a closer look at fat and learn…

Why Fat Is the Key to Good Health

Contrary to the nutritional "wisdom" most of us get from the media and food packaging, not all fat is bad for you. In fact, your body needs a certain amount of fat to nourish cells, supply essential fatty acids, and to trigger the release of a hormone that signals your brain that you are full. Fat also slows down the conversion of carbohydrates into glucose, feeding your brain a steady flow of glucose, not a sudden rush that triggers an excess insulin response.

Most importantly, eating the *right kind* of fat is the key to boosting your immune system and staying healthy. That's because certain fats provide linoleic acid, the raw material that your body needs to produce amazing microhormones called *eicosanoids*.

... eating the right kind of fat is the key to boosting your immune system and staying healthy.

The body of knowledge about eicosanoids is a new, exciting and ever expanding area of scientific research. Think of eicosanoids as master control hormones that regulate many of your body's biological functions, including other hormones such as insulin and glucagon.

Your body manufactures two families of eicosanoids — Good eicosanoids (known as Series One) and Bad eicosanoids (Series Two).

Good Series-One Eicosanoids	Bad Series-Two Eicosanoids
Enhance immunity	Suppress immunity
Decrease inflammation	Increase inflammation
Decrease pain	Increase pain
Increase oxygen flow	Decrease oxygen flow
Increase endurance	Decrease endurance
Prevent blood clotting	Promote blood clotting
Dilate airways	Constrict airways
Increase rate of cell growth	Decrease rate of cell growth

Note: Once again, "bad" is a relative term. For example, while "bad" eicosanoids may constrict blood vessels and airways, they also promote blood clotting, which stops you from bleeding to death from a paper cut.

Leading researchers continue to explore the link between the kinds of eicosanoids the body manufactures and wellness. Evidence continues to mount that poor health and disease may be due to your body making more "bad" eicosanoids than "good" eicosanoids. In other words, the key to good health is to produce more good eicosanoids than bad eicosanoids.

The good news is that the kind of eicosanoids your body manufactures are largely dependent on the food you eat. And this is why following a strict low-fat diet is no guarantee of better health.

The Total Health eating program will help you achieve a balance of good and bad eicosanoids that will boost your immune system and stay healthy. Here's how...

Three Steps to Improve Your Eicosanoid Balance

1. Eat protein-rich, favorable-carbohydrate meals. As you know, following the Total Health eating program stimulates the release of fat-burning glucagon and inhibits the release of fat-storing insulin. These same powerful hormones also affect the production of good and bad eicosanoids. Insulin activates delta 5 desaturase, an enzyme that promotes the production of bad eicosanoids. Glucagon, which works in opposition to insulin, inhibits this enzyme.

Excess carbohydrates also inhibit another important enzyme called delta 6 desaturase. Delta 6 desaturase allows linoleic acid — the raw material your body needs to make all eicosanoids — to enter the eicosanoid production pathway. When this enzyme is active, your body processes all the linoleic acid it needs to produce eicosanoids.

Eating more protein and less carbohydrates is the most important step you can take to restore your eicosanoid balance.

2. Eat foods that supply plenty of linoleic acid. Linoleic acid is the essential fatty acid that your body uses as building blocks for all eicosanoids. Without adequate amounts of linoleic acid, you are starving your body's eicosanoid production pipeline. The best food sources for linoleic acid are olive, almond, hazelnut, safflower, light sesame, sunflower and walnut oils.

3. Stay away from trans fatty acids. Trans fatty acids are found in oils with fats that have been altered by food manufacturers. Trans fatty acids inhibit the delta 6 desaturase enzyme and the production of good eicosanoids. They have also been linked to heart disease.

... go back to putting butter on your vegetables. Butter is not that bad for you.

One of the most common sources of trans fatty acids is partially hydrogenated vegetable oil, the key ingredient in margarine, processed peanut butter and thousands of other food products. So look for natural peanut butter (the kind with the oil on top) and go back to putting butter on your vegetables. Butter is not that bad for you.

Don't mistake my recommendation to use butter as a license to go wild. To make the Total Health program work, you need to eat the right kinds of fat in the right amount. See your customized menu choices for more information.

More Ways to Make Good Eicosanoids

For most people, eating protein-rich, favorable-carbohydrate meals, fats rich in linoleic acid and avoiding foods loaded with trans fatty acids is enough to kick the production of good eicosanoids into high gear. But to tip the odds even more in your favor, here are three more ways to fine tune your balance of eicosanoids:

• **Avoid foods with high levels of alpha linoleic acid (ALA).** ALA is another fatty acid that suppresses good eicosanoid production by inhibiting the delta 6 desaturase enzyme. ALA is primarily found in flaxseed oil, soybean oil and canola oil. Instead, use olive oil, which has no ALA. If the distinctive taste of olive oil is a problem, another good choice is light sesame oil.

• **Watch your intake of arachidonic acid (AA).** This fatty acid is found in the fat of red meat, organ meats and egg yolks. Your body converts AA directly into bad eicosanoids. If you choose to eat red meat, trim off the fat to avoid the fat's high AA content. Instead of egg yolks, use egg whites or egg substitutes.

Watching the amount of arachidonic acid you ingest is only important if you are overly sensitive to large amounts. Signs of AA sensitivity include brittle hair and nails, dry, flaking skin and minor rashes. If you are reducing excess insulin and producing more glucagon and you are not experiencing these symptoms, you probably don't have a problem with AA.

• **Eat foods rich in eicosapentaenoic acid (EPA).** EPA is an essential fatty acid found in fish oil that slows the production of bad eicosanoids. Good sources of EPA include salmon, tuna, herring and fish oil capsules.

Putting It All Together

Okay, we've talked about the connection between the food you eat, your blood sugar level and the hormonal response to burn or store body fat. How does this work in the real world?

To get started on a protein-rich, favorable-carbohydrate way of eating, the first thing you have to do is figure out your daily protein requirement. In other words, how much protein you are supposed to have during the course of a day.

Your daily protein requirement is determined by your percentage of lean body mass. Lean body mass refers to the percentage of your body that isn't fat, which is made up of muscle, bone and your organs. The fastest and most accurate way to determine your lean body mass is to use an electrical impedance body fat analyzer like the one I use for my patients.

Another factor which determines how much protein you need is your body frame size. For instance, if you have a large body frame you need between 90 to 100 grams of protein per day.

Exactly how many grams of carbohydrate you need is determined by your percentage of body fat and weight.

For example, if you're at your ideal body fat and weight, you can eat a one-to-one ratio of protein to carbohydrate. Again, if you have a large body frame, that is 100 grams of protein to 100 grams of carbohydrate per day.

If you want moderate weight loss of 2 to 3 pounds a week or about 10 pounds a month, you would still eat 100 grams of protein per day. But you would limit yourself to about 40 grams of carbs a day. That's roughly a 2 to 1 ratio of protein to carbohydrate.

> This protein-rich diet signals your body to release fat-burning, good eicosanoid-building glucagon and keeps fat-storing, bad eicosanoid-building insulin in check.

Timing Is Everything

The key to regulating your blood sugars and burning body fat consistently is to eat every 3½ to 4 hours.

Remember the idea that food is a drug? One key to using drugs effectively is to make sure you take your medicine at regular intervals to maintain an even dosage level. The same principle applies to the Total Health eating program.

The key to regulating your blood sugars and burning body fat consistently is to eat every 3½ to 4 hours. This interval promotes optimal metabolism and blood sugar regulation. So I put my patients on a schedule of breakfast at 8 a.m., lunch around noon, a snack around 3:30 in the afternoon, dinner around 7 p.m., and an optional bedtime snack around 11 p.m.

Here's how your daily protein and carbohydrate requirements are portioned out over the course of a day:

28 grams of protein at breakfast, lunch and dinner and 7 grams at the afternoon and night-time snack for a total of 98 grams protein.

10 grams of carbs at breakfast, lunch and dinner and 5 grams at the afternoon and night time snack for a total of 40 grams carbohydrate.

Breakfast/Lunch/Dinner	Two Snacks	Total
28 g Protein	7 g Protein	98 g Protein
10 g Carbs	5 g Carbs	40 g Carbs

Typical Total Health Menu Options

Here are some sample Total Health menu options to show you how easy it is to follow the Total Health eating program in the real world. An extensive list of foods and menu options is provided to all Total Health patients. These food lists and menus are also available at our Web site: **www.totalhealthdoc.com**

Sample Breakfast Option
• Omelette with Cheese, Meat
   Mushrooms, Onions and Avocado
   — and —
• Favorite Fruit or Tomatoes

Sample Lunch or Dinner Options
• Chicken, Fish or Meat with Veggies
• Avocado Stuffed with Tuna Salad
• Chinese Chicken Salad

Sample Fast Food Options
• McDonald's Egg McMuffin (open-faced)
• Double Cheeseburger (open-faced or wrapped in lettuce)

Sample Snack Options
• Celery Stalk with Peanut Butter
• Cheese Stick with Fruit
• ¼ Cup of Nuts
• Caffe Latte Coffee Drink

How Do You Count Fat?

Don't worry about fat. The concept of counting units of fat tends to confuse people. The Total Health program provides all the fat you need automatically from the protein-rich, favorable-carbohydrate food choices that you make.

The Total Health program provides all the fat you need automatically from the protein-rich, favorable-carbohydrate food choices that you make.

Remember, it's not the fat you eat that raises your cholesterol. It's the excess insulin from all those carbohydrates you've been eating. For a lot of people, this is hard to believe.

Until I show them the hard proof...

On the following pages are actual blood tests from one of my patients. The first one was done through his M.D. It showed a triglyceride level at 361, twice the high end of normal, which is between 50 and 190. Cholesterol was at 268. Normal is at 130 to 200 (see Blood Test #1).

Blood Test #1: Before Total Health

GREGORY H. JOHNSON, M.D.
227 W. JANSS RD., SUITE 215
THOUSAND OAKS, CA 91360
TELEPHONE (805) 497-0597

LABORATORY REPORT

TECH

PATIENT: 19906

CH10 HEP AMYL THYROI

SEX:
ROOM:
DR.   JOHNSON

AGE:
DATE DRAWN: 08-27-96

COMMENTS:

TEST	RESULT		FLAGS	NORMAL RANGE	DATE RUN	LO NORM HI
GLUCOSE	80	MG/DL		65 - 110	08-27-96	
BUN	20	MG/DL		7 - 22		
CREATININE	0.9	MG/DL		0.5 - 1.5		
URIC ACID	3.6	MG/DL		2.5 - 7.7		
TRIGLYCERIDES	361	MG/DL	HIGH	50 - 190		
CHOLESTEROL	266	MG/DL	HIGH	130 - 200		
T. PROTEIN	8.1	G/DL	HIGH	6.2 - 8.0		
ALBUMIN	4.8	G/DL		3.8 - 5.1		
T. BILIRUBIN	1.2	MG/DL		0.1 - 1.2		
AST (SGOT)	27	IU/L		8 - 41		
ALT (SGPT)	35	IU/L		8 - 40		
LDH	127	IU/L		80 - 194		
ALK PHOS	69	IU/L		35 - 123		
GGT	23	IU/L		0 - 45		
SODIUM	140.2	MEQ/L		135.0 - 150.0		
POTASSIUM	3.68	MEQ/L		3.50 - 5.30		
CHLORIDE	100	MEQ/L		95 - 105		
AMYLASE	23	U/L		0 - 96		
AMYLASE	23	U/L		0 - 96		

10-31-96
CHOLESTEROL   289
TRIGLYCERIDES 561
HDL   32
CHOL/HDL RISK
RATIO   9.0   ELEVATED CORONARY HEART DISEASE (CHD) RISK
(6.7-14.3)

Patient informed
Date 8-27-96
Initial

AUG 27 1996

Obviously, his physician was quite alarmed, so he ran another blood test a couple months later. Now his cholesterol was at 289; triglycerides were up to 561. His HDLs were at 32, so his cholesterol to HDL or high density lipid risk ratio was 9.0. That's well within the elevated coronary heart disease risk category. In other words, he was a heart attack waiting to happen. And he was just 44 years old.

Blood Test #2: After Total Health

After seven weeks on the Total Health program, my patient had dropped 30 pounds. His cholesterol went from 289 to 174, which is within the normal range. His triglycerides went from 561 down to 107, which is smack in the middle of normal. His cholesterol to HDL ratio or his heart disease risk ratio went from 9.0 to 3.7, which is below average risk.

These results astonished my patient — and his coworkers. For months, they watched this guy eat double cheeseburgers wrapped in lettuce for lunch. They thought he was nuts. But the numbers on these blood tests don't lie.

Part 2: Micronutrients

If you're like most Americans, chances are you've got at least one — and probably several — half-full bottles of vitamin and mineral supplements in your medicine cabinet.

And no wonder. It seems every day some new study or article or health guru says Vitamin X or Mineral Y helps you stay healthy or prevent some horrible disease. Then every other day, a new study or article or guru says the stuff you just bought is no good. Worse, Vitamin X can actually cause a different, but equally horrible disease. Besides, what you really need is Vitamin Z!

Thanks to an increasingly health conscious public and relentless marketing, sales of vitamins and other nutritional supplements have skyrocketed! According to the Council for Responsible Nutrition, a trade group for the supplement industry, an estimated 100 million Americans are spending $6.5 billion a year on vitamins, minerals and nutritional supplements. That's up from $3 billion in 1990.

Two factors are driving the explosive growth in supplement sales. First, as Baby Boomers get older, more and more people are becoming active participants in their own health care. This consumer health care movement is being fueled by easier access to medical information and acceptance of health care options such as acupuncture and chiropractic by traditional medical organizations.

The other reason for all the marketing hype about nutritional supplements is the Dietary Supplement Health and Education Act of 1994. This law allows supplement makers to market their products as "dietary supplements" and thus avoid the scientific scrutiny and expense of the FDA prescription drug review process. As long as supplement manufacturers do not claim their products offer specific health benefits, they are free to sell their wares over the counter, through mail order and over the Internet.

Confused?

The following pages will help you sort through the hype. We'll start with a brief review of vitamin and mineral fundamentals. Then we'll take a closer look at how vitamin and mineral supplements, water and fiber contribute to optimal health.

Vitamin and Mineral Basics

Micronutrients — commonly known as vitamins and minerals — perform a number of essential functions to help your body grow, convert food into energy and stay healthy.

Vitamins are organic and allow your body to process carbohydrates, proteins and fats. They also act as catalysts by triggering or speeding up chemical reactions. There are a total of 13 vitamins, which nutritionists classify into two groups. Four vitamins — A, D, E and K — are called "fat-soluble" because they are stored in your body's fat. They are usually found together in the fats and oils of food.

The other nine are "water-soluble" and are not stored in large amounts in your body. The water-soluble vitamins include vitamin C and the eight B vitamins — thiamine (B-1), riboflavin (B-2), niacin (B-3), pyridoxine (B-6), pantothenic acid, cyanocobalamin (B-12), biotin and folic acid (folate).

Minerals are inorganic substances that promote a variety of important biochemical processes. There are 15 dietary minerals, which nutritionists also classify into two groups: Major minerals are needed in amounts greater than 100 milligrams a day. Trace minerals are needed in amounts less than 100 milligrams a day.

The major minerals include calcium, phosphorus, magnesium, sodium, chloride, potassium and sulfur. The trace minerals include iron, iodine, copper, chromium, fluoride, manganese, molybdenum, selenium and zinc.

How Much Do You Need?

When it comes to taking vitamins and mineral supplements, the question of "how much?" is a source of continuing controversy.

Most established medical, scientific and nutritional sources say you get all the vitamins and minerals you need from eating a balanced diet. Follow the general nutritional guidelines such as the Recommended Dietary Allowances (RDAs) and you'll be fine.

The Balanced Diet Problem

Do you eat a balanced diet? Do you know anyone who does? That's the big problem with the notion that the food you eat provides all the vitamins and minerals you need. Most Americans don't eat the wide variety of food necessary to obtain the right amount of the micronutrients they need.

For example, in a study published in the *New England Journal of Medicine* in March 1998, researchers from the Harvard Medical School estimated that 40 percent of Americans may have Vitamin D deficiencies. Forty percent!

Our rushed, junk food, no-time-for-breakfast or lunch, prepackaged, processed, frozen-food culture does not encourage a balanced diet. And as you know, if you're not eating the right balance of foods in the right amount, vitamin and mineral deficiencies may be the least of your problems! No multivitamin supplement will compensate for lousy eating habits.

Are the RDAs Enough?

Since 1941, the Food and Nutrition Board of the Institute of Medicine, National Academy of Sciences, has set RDAs to recommend the minimum amount of vitamins and minerals needed to prevent diseases caused by vitamin and mineral deficiencies.

For years, this approach has been criticized by a growing and increasingly vocal number of respected medical researchers and doctors. They argue that the intake levels dictated by the RDAs are just enough to help you survive, not thrive. Instead, vitamins and minerals should be taken in amounts that

Our rushed junk food, no-time-for-breakfast or lunch, prepackaged, processed, frozen-food culture does not encourage a balanced diet.

prevent chronic diseases and promote optimal health, a state in which your body functions at its best.

It's taken some time, but the government nutrition experts, the folks who set the official nutritional standards, are catching up. Slowly but surely, RDAs are being reset to recommend higher amounts of specific vitamins and minerals.

In 1997, the Board announced that the RDAs were now just one part of an expanded set of nutritional guidelines called Dietary Reference Intakes (DRIs). The DRIs reflect the latest scientific consensus on the role vitamins and minerals play in optimum health. For example, the first DRI report, on calcium, revised intake levels upwards to prevent bone loss caused by osteoporosis instead of just preventing a calcium deficiency.

New DRIs on folate and other B vitamins were published in 1998. As funding becomes available, new DRIs — which will include updated and expanded RDAs — will be set for other nutrient groups, including antioxidants, macronutrients, trace minerals, and fiber.

As nutritional research becomes more influential in mainstream medicine, it's now routine for M.D.s to prescribe high doses of vitamins and minerals to address specific conditions or diseases. For example, high doses of calcium are often prescribed for women to prevent osteoporosis. High doses of folic acid are often prescribed for women as part of good pre- and post-natal care. People who suffer from anemia usually need iron supplements.

The Total Health Approach to Vitamins and Minerals

1. Eat a protein-rich, favorable-carbohydrate diet. The best way to make sure your body is supplied with a continuing source of essential micronutrients is to eat a wide variety of foods. It bears repeating that no vitamin or mineral supplement can compensate for the benefits of eating a properly balanced protein-rich, favorable-carbohydrate diet. That's why they're called vitamin and mineral supplements — not replacements.

2. Do no harm! Do not take megadoses of vitamins or minerals unless prescribed by your doctor to treat a specific deficiency. Some vitamin advocates go so far as to recommend massive doses of certain vitamins to ward off ailments ranging from cancer to impotence. The FDA and mainstream medicine regard these perpetual vitamin fads as quackery — and often dangerous. For example, large amounts of vitamin A can contribute to liver damage. Excess doses of vitamin D can contribute to kidney damage. Iron, zinc, chromium and selenium can be toxic at just five times the RDA. The most common cause of poisoning deaths among children is adult-strength iron supplements.

> **... no vitamin or mineral supplement can compensate for the benefits of eating a properly balanced protein-rich, favorable-carbohydrate diet.**

3. Use vitamin and mineral supplements as nutritional insurance. The Total Health program provides your body with the essential micronutrients it needs from two sources: the food you eat and a high-quality vitamin and mineral supplement.

How to Choose the Right Vitamin and Mineral Supplement

High-quality supplements generally contain the following vitamins and minerals. If you are confused about what kind of supplement to purchase, you may want to consider our Total Health Pack Morning and Evening Formula. Total Health Pack contains an essential blend of vitamins, minerals, herbs and fiber. It's custom-designed to enhance the effectiveness of your Total Health program.

Antioxidants

Antioxidants counter the harmful effects of a chemical chain reaction caused by free radicals. Free radicals are chemically reactive oxygen molecules that are missing an electron. Because electrons prefer to travel in pairs, free radicals aggressively steal electrons from healthy molecules. The electron-stealing chain reaction that results produces compounds that cause cellular damage.

Antioxidants counter the harmful effects of a chemical chain reaction caused by free radicals.

Free radicals are a natural byproduct of cell metabolism, the process by which cells use oxygen to create energy. Exposure to everyday environmental factors such as cigarette smoke, air pollution and sunlight also stimulate free radical production.

Scientists estimate that each cell in the body may get pounded with as many as 10,000 free radical hits a day! Your body does its best to counter free radicals naturally, but over time free radical build up takes its toll. It's no wonder that many scientists link free radical damage to cancer, heart disease, cataracts and premature aging.

Antioxidants counter free radical damage by supplying extra electrons that bind with and stabilize free radical molecules. Antioxidant-rich foods and supplements provide the body with the ammunition it needs to fend off the non-stop free radical bombardment.

Some of the most commonly known antioxidant nutrients are vitamins A, C and E.

Phytonutrients

Phytonutrients or phytochemicals are nutrients from plants that promote a variety of beneficial functions. Many exhibit powerful antioxidant properties. Scientists are working feverishly to mine the largely unexplored potential that phytonutrients hold for medicine. Some of the research has revealed amazing possibilities.

One class of phytonutrient found in grape seeds, for example, exhibits antioxidant properties for up to three days in the body. More importantly, it is able to cross the blood-brain barrier. Brain tissue is particularly susceptible to free radical-induced oxidation. This phytonutrient also inhibits enzymes that break down vitamins C and E into less useful nutrients.

Some of the best phytonutrients are proanthocyanidins (grape seed extract), sulforaphane (broccoli extract), and lycopene (tomato extract).

Chelated Minerals and Trace Elements

Dietary minerals and trace elements support necessary biochemical processes that help your body burn fat, build muscle, strengthen bones, promote healing and deliver oxygen to the cells.

Proper absorption or bioavailability is essential for effective mineral and trace element supplementation. Minerals and trace elements are more rapidly absorbed by the intestinal tract when they are chelated — or wrapped — in an amino acid coating. Chelated calcium, for example, is absorbed 60 times more effectively than the calcium in milk.

Enzymes

All biochemical reactions are started or accelerated by a special class of protein molecules called enzymes. One of the best known enzyme supplements is lactase, which helps people who are lactose intolerant or unable to properly digest dairy products.

Bromelain is another enzyme getting a lot of attention for its digestive benefits. It's found in particularly high concentrations in pineapple. Bromelain is also being studied for its therapeutic value in treating severe bruises, inflammation and soft tissue injuries.

Pancreatic enzymes such as amylase, protease and lipase are also used to treat malabsorption syndromes, when the body's ability to digest a variety of nutrients is greatly impaired.

Herbs

The Total Health Pack supplements also contain herbal extracts to enhance your health, including ginseng and ginkgo biloba.

Ginseng, a staple of Chinese herbal medicine, stimulates the adrenal and pituitary glands to increase energy and resistance to stress. Total Health Pack uses American ginseng. The Chinese variety is a more powerful stimulant and is not recommended for use if you have high blood pressure.

Ginkgo biloba has been used by the Chinese for thousands of years. Recent medical research has heralded ginkgo biloba's ability to increase blood flow to the brain, which helps boost memory and mental acuity.

Got Water?

Why You Need to Drink More

Are you drinking enough water? If you're like most of my patients, the answer is not as much as you know you should.

Water helps your body digest food, absorb nutrients, and transport those nutrients throughout your body. It's also a vital part of your body's waste removal system. Without adequate amounts of water, your body becomes dehydrated and cannot function properly. More acute cases of dehydration can cause fatigue, nausea and dementia. Severe cases often lead to heat exhaustion, heat stroke and even death.

... most of us live in a habitual state of mild dehydration.

You don't have to run for hours in the summer sun to become dehydrated. In fact, most of us live in a habitual state of mild dehydration. Sure, we drink water every day, but it's not enough. Or, we think that drinking water-based fluids, such as coffee, tea or soda, is the same as drinking water. It's not. Coffee, tea and many sodas contain caffeine, a diuretic that dehydrates your body.

Make no mistake. Dehydration, however mild, can lead to serious health problems. If you aren't drinking enough water, over time your kidneys will pay the price. Your kidneys are an integral part of your body's purification system. Their main job is to clean your blood of toxins and metabolic wastes. And to function properly, they rely on a steady and sufficient flow of water.

The less water you drink, the more stress your kidneys suffer, and the less efficient they become. Over time, this chronic abuse can contribute to escalating health problems, ranging from increased likeliness of illness to painful kidney stones to kidney failure.

The bottom line: If you've been blessed with two good kidneys, take care of them by drinking plenty of water.

Flush Away Excess Body Fat

Drinking lots of water doesn't wash away body fat, but it does help your kidneys flush out the metabolic waste that is generated by burning excess body fat. Some of this waste is partially burned fat which passes from your body in stool or urine. So the more water you drink, the more urine you generate, and the more fat your body gets rid of.

... the more water you drink ... the more fat your body gets rid of.

How Much Water Do You Need?

The general medical consensus is about two quarts or six to eight glasses a day. You need even more if you exercise regularly or live in a hot climate.

The Best Way to Monitor Your Water Intake

Don't watch the amount of liquid going into your body. Watch the liquid that's going out. Take note of the frequency and color of your urine. As a general rule, you're drinking enough if you urinate regularly and the color is clear or a pale yellow. If you urinate infrequently or the color is a bright or dark yellow, your body needs more water.

Water and Total Health

Here's another reason to drink enough water...

Along with storing fat, excess insulin levels also promote water retention. As your Total Health program stabilizes your insulin levels, you'll start to shed this excess water. To stay hydrated, you need to replenish your body's water supply.

Drinking the right amount of water every day may take some practice. Here are some tips to get you in the hydration habit...

• **Start your day with an eight-ounce glass of water.** Your body is always dehydrated after six to eight hours without water. The sooner you hydrate, the better and more alert you'll feel — before that first cup of coffee!

• **Drink an eight-ounce glass before breakfast, lunch and dinner.** Water before meals tends to take an edge off hunger.

- **Reduce your consumption of coffee and other caffeinated beverages to one or two cups a day.** Aside from its diuretic quality, coffee can also stimulate excess insulin production. Replace those extra cups of coffee with hot water. Add lemon for flavor, if you like. Herbal teas are also okay. Many people have discovered that sipping hot water or herbal tea is a remarkably effective way to wean themselves off caffeine. Reduce your caffeine consumption gradually to minimize the headaches and mood swings that often accompany caffeine withdrawal.

- **Ask yourself if you're thirsty**. Chances are you're much more thirsty than you realize. Asking the question forces you to become aware of your thirst. But you can't do anything about it unless you have water on hand. When water is out of sight, it's out of mind. That's why you should…

- **Take water with you.** Next time you're in the grocery story, buy a flat of 16-ounce disposable water bottles. Take one with you wherever you go…in the car, at work, on errands, when you go for a walk. When the bottle is empty, refill it. One way to keep track of your water intake is to place four rubber bands around the bottle. Each time you finish 16 ounces, take off a rubber band.

- **Get bubbly.** These days, supermarkets have entire aisles dedicated to bottled water products. For variety, put some plain or flavored carbonated water in your cart. Look for orange, lemon or lime flavored sparkling water. Stay away from carbonated water flavored with juice. You want the bubbles, not the extra sugar.

• **Monitor your water output.** The best indication that you're drinking more water is that you are urinating more frequently. Do not think of this as an inconvenience. Think of it as a sign that you are doing your part to help your body's natural purification system keep you healthy.

Fiber Facts

Let's do a little word association. If I say "fiber" — what's the first thought that pops into your head?

If you said "constipation," you're being honest. Most of us think of fiber as the stuff that keeps our bowels "regular" — what mom and dad used to refer to less delicately as "roughage."

What Is Fiber?

Fiber is the part of plant food that your body can't digest.

Actually, there are five different kinds of fiber. Nutritionists divide them into two main categories: soluble and insoluble fiber.

• **The soluble fibers are pectin and gum.** They are found in foods such as beans, oats and citrus fruits. Soluble fibers dissolve and thicken in water.

• **The insoluble fibers are cellulose, hemicellulose and lignin.** They are found in foods such as wheat bran, nuts, seeds and fruits. Insoluble fibers include the outer coating of grains and the skins of fruits and vegetables. Insoluble fibers do not dissolve in water.

Why Fiber Is Good for You

Fiber diminishes the body's insulin response.

Thanks to increasing scientific study, fiber is getting a lot more respect than it's well-deserved reputation as a natural remedy for constipation. The medical community now recognizes fiber as an essential dietary component with long-term health benefits.

- **Fiber helps prevent hemorrhoids.** Hemorrhoids are the painful swelling of veins near the anus most often caused by strained bowel movements. Fiber softens and adds bulk to bowel movements, making them easier to pass.

- **Fiber reduces the risk of heart disease by lowering cholesterol levels.** Fiber binds to cholesterol and evacuates it in the stool before its absorption into the blood stream.

- **Fiber helps regulate insulin levels.** Fiber diminishes the body's insulin response by inhibiting the absorption of glucose into the blood stream.

- **Fiber may reduce the risk of certain cancers.** For years, researchers have said that high-fiber diets may reduce the risk of colon, rectal and breast cancer. A number of explanations have been offered. One popular theory holds that fiber speeds up the passage of harmful waste through the intestines, minimizing their absorption and contact with intestinal cells.

How Much Fiber Do You Need?

The general medical consensus is between 25 and 40 grams daily. Most Americans get less than half that amount. That's why your Total Health program makes it easy to get all the fiber you need. You just don't get it from carbohydrate-loaded food choices that stimulate excess insulin production and fat storage.

On the Total Health program you can get your fiber — even when you go against the grain…

- **Choose your carbohydrates in the form of fiber-rich fruits and vegetables.** For a list of fruits and vegetables that qualify as fiber-rich carbohydrates, see your custom Total Health menu.

- **If you must eat bread or pasta, limit the amount** and choose whole grains.

- **Take your Total Health Pack nutritional supplements.** It complements your protein-rich, favorable-carbohydrate eating program with a variety of fibers, including grapefruit fiber, apple pectin, pysillium husk, oat bran, guar gum, barley bran and pineapple stem.

- **Take a fiber supplement,** such as Metamucil or Rexall's Bios Life.

A final tip: Increase your fiber intake gradually! Too much fiber can cause gas or diarrhea. To avoid these natural side effects, drink plenty of water.

4

Exercise:
How to Get Started and Why

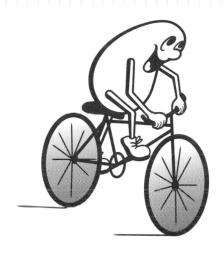

Not getting enough exercise? You're not alone. The number of Americans whose idea of physical activity is reaching for the remote control has reached crisis proportions.

In 1996, a U.S. Surgeon General's report estimated that 60 percent of adult Americans were not physically active on a regular basis. And 25 percent of adults — that's one in four Americans — were not active at all! In 1999, a follow up survey conducted for a non-profit weight loss support group reported that nearly half (48%) of Americans claimed to exercise regularly.

That figure — while encouraging — still leaves more than half of American adults on the couch. Is it any wonder that the number of people who are disabled or killed by obesity-related diseases grows every year?

If you are serious about living in total health, you must make regular physical activity part of your life. In this chapter, we'll take a look at how your body *and mind* benefit from a combination of aerobic, resistance and passive exercise. You'll also learn insider tips on choosing a health club and working with a personal trainer.

Why Exercise Is Important

The benefits of regular physical activity are astounding. For starters, exercise increases your metabolism to help you burn fat. Exercise boosts your stamina, strength and flexibility. It strengthens bones and improves your posture. And it lowers your risk of heart disease, high blood pressure, stroke and diabetes.

The benefits of regular physical activity are astounding.

Physical activity also increases your self-esteem and confidence. You'll look better and you'll feel better about the way you look. It reduces stress, improves your mood and helps you sleep better. New research also suggests that exercise may even stimulate brain cell growth and slow the aging process.

Your body needs to move. If you don't use it, losing it is just a matter of time. As you get older, even simple tasks like climbing stairs will leave your lungs winded and your heart racing. Your joints will stiffen and your bones will weaken. Injuries will occur more often — with more serious consequences. Your range of motion will also suffer. You'll have to watch the way you bend over to pick up the paper. Turning your neck to back your car out of the driveway will be a struggle.

If you doubt me, I suggest you spend a day in a retirement community. Talk to people who've learned about the importance of regular exercise the hard way. They'll tell you that no matter how busy you are, it's a lot easier — and a lot less painful — to work with a personal trainer now, rather than a chiropractor or physical therapist later.

How Regular Exercise Burns Fat Faster

After more than 1,000 Total Health consultations, I noticed that some of my patients made consistently faster progress towards their goals. What were these "fast track" patients doing differently? The "secret" was remarkably simple…

Clients who lost weight faster — and kept it off — made exercise a regular part of their weekly routine!

… your body has a powerful hormonal response to exercise.

While it's true that many Total Health patients lose weight just by eating protein-rich, favorable-carbohydrate meals, following a regular exercise program turbocharges your body's ability to burn fat. Here's how…

First, exercise boosts your metabolism — the complex biochemical process by which food is converted into energy. The lower your metabolic rate, the harder it is for you to burn calories. The faster your metabolic rate, the easier it is to lose weight. More about how to speed up your metabolism in a moment.

Second —and more importantly — your body has a powerful hormonal response to exercise.

Aerobic exercise, such as jogging, bicycling and swimming, stimulates the release of glucagon — the fat burning hormone — and inhibits the release of insulin — the fat storage hormone.

Resistance exercise, such as weight training, stimulates the release of human growth hormone — which burns fat and helps rebuild muscle.

... following a regular exercise program turbocharges your body's ability to burn fat.

When you follow your Total Health eating program *and* commit to a regular exercise routine, your body becomes a fat-burning machine. Thanks to your body's hormonal response to a protein-rich, favorable-carbohydrate diet, your high glucagon levels are already mobilizing stored fat to be burned as energy. Burning body fat gives you more than twice the amount of energy than burning sugars. The result is more energy for your workout.

The complete opposite is true when you "carbo-load" before a workout. Carbohydrates stimulate the release of insulin and inhibit the release of glucagon. Your workout is fueled by sugar, not stored body fat.

There is another benefit of high glucagon levels prior to exercise. Glucagon helps widen blood vessels, allowing your muscles access to more oxygen and nutrients. The result is a better workout and a faster recovery.

There are two basic types of active exercise: aerobic and resistance. If you want to lose unwanted body fat and gain lean fat-burning muscle mass, you need to do both.

Aerobic Exercise

Aerobic exercise works your heart and lungs to improve your body's ability to use oxygen as an energy source. The goal is to increase your stamina by training your body to work more efficiently and use less energy to do the same amount of work. The sooner your heart rate and breathing return to resting levels after a workout, the better your conditioning.

Aerobic activities are continuous and rhythmic, such as walking, hiking, jogging, bicycling and swimming. To benefit from aerobic exercise, you need to exercise at 60 to 80 percent of your maximum heart rate for 20 to 30 minutes at least three times a week. To figure out your maximum heart rate, subtract your age from 220.

There are two ways to measure your heartbeats per minute. One way is to count your pulse beats for 15 seconds, then multiply that number by four. The other is to invest in a heart rate monitor. Models vary in sophistication, from about $75 to more than $200.

Resistance Exercise

Pumping iron may seem like a mindless activity, but your body gains tremendous benefits. Resistance exercise or weight training builds your muscular strength, endurance, definition and tone. In the process, it also develops stronger bones and improves your posture. Most importantly, lifting weights accelerates your metabolism.

How many times have you heard someone say that the reason they can't lose weight is because they have a slow metabolism? Or listen to someone explain that the reason they never gain weight is a naturally fast metabolism? The implication is that your metabolic rate — fast or slow — is a matter of genetic fate and out of your control.

Resistance exercise fuels your body's natural fat-burning cycle.

That's just not true. Metabolism is a function of muscle mass. If you have the metabolism of a napping snail, it's because you have a low ratio of muscle tissue to fat tissue.

This is why resistance exercise using resistance bands or weights must be part of your workout routine. The more lean muscle mass you have, the higher your metabolism. The faster your metabolism, the easier it is for your body to burn — and avoid storing — fat. Even when you're resting!

Resistance exercise tears down muscle fiber, which stimulates the pituitary gland to release human growth hormone. Human growth hormone is broadly recognized by the scientific and medical community as one of the body's most powerful hormones. Longevity experts believe it may be the key to reversing the affects of aging. It's also known as a ferocious fat-burner.

Human growth hormone mobilizes stored body fat to strained muscles, where it is burned as energy to repair torn muscle fiber. It's during this healing process that muscles gain bulk, tone and definition.

Resistance exercise fuels your body's natural fat-burning cycle. Human growth hormone burns more fat and builds more muscle, which makes it even easier for your body to burn more fat. And every time you lift weights, this amazing process repeats itself!

And you thought pumping iron was just for guys named Moose!

Passive Exercise

Passive exercise is essential for proper muscle and joint health. It increases your flexibility or your ability to bend, stretch and twist easily. It improves your balance and coordination, and it reduces your risk of injury. Regular passive exercise may even slow the progression of osteoarthritis and other degenerative joint conditions.

There are two kinds of passive exercise: Do-it-yourself stretching exercises and the muscle and joint mobilization performed by a qualified healthcare professional, such as a doctor of chiropractic. As you age, muscle stretching and joint mobilization will help preserve and improve your mobility and range of motion.

Maintaining mobility is one of the keys to longevity and aging gracefully.

Stretching before and after workouts will help you avoid pulled muscles, cramps and a variety of other injuries. It will also speed your recovery. Moist heat and a skilled massage or physical therapist can do wonders to loosen knots and tight muscles.

Your joints also need special attention. As you age, calcium salts seep into the joints, causing accelerated wear much the same way sand wears down gears in a machine. This contributes to a condition called osteoarthritis, which over time, often leads to restricted movement.

Maintaining mobility is one of the keys to longevity and aging gracefully. Many entertainment and sports celebrities have extended their careers and preserved their range of motion well into their seventies and eighties thanks to periodic massage and joint mobilization.

Think of all the preventive maintenance it takes to keep your car running. Oil changes every 3,000 miles. New tires every 50,000 miles. A new timing belt around 75,000. Not to mention all the spark plugs, filters and fluids that are replaced according to the service schedule.

You understand that if you don't take care of your car it's only a matter of time before it breaks down for good.

Now if money is no obstacle and you just can't be bothered with maintenance, when your car stops running, you can just go out and buy another. There are plenty of cars in the world.

The human body is the most complicated machine in the world — and you only get one of them. If you want to get the most from yours, take care of it. Give yourself the fuel you need. Exercise. And put yourself on a regular joint maintenance schedule. In the long run, you'll find it's a lot easier — and less expensive — to stay healthy than to keep your car running, anyway.

Choosing a Health Club

Choosing to start an exercise program is easy. Making exercise part of a lifelong commitment to fitness is another matter. The key is to schedule a regular time for exercise and then stick to your schedule until exercise becomes a habit. For most people, the *minimum* amount of time it takes to develop a natural exercise habit is six weeks. That's one-hour of focused exercise, three times a week for six weeks.

Too many people start exercising filled with unrealistic goals and expectations. And when they don't see dramatic weight loss, rock hard abs or "buns of steel" after a couple weeks, they get discouraged. They procrastinate. They get distracted by other priorities. Before long, they're back on the couch.

If you are serious about living in Total Health, and you want to make exercise part of your lifestyle, consider joining a health club. There are a number of advantages...

• **Focus and Motivation.** Once you're at the health club, you've overcome the number one obstacle to sticking with a regular exercise program: showing up. Now, you have no more excuses. You're not distracted by the phone, the laundry, the kids or a myriad of household chores. You are there to work out. And so is most everyone else. It's really hard to procrastinate when everyone around you is in motion.

• **Equipment Choices.** Good health clubs invest in a variety of top-quality aerobic and resistance training equipment.

You'll find several ways to get an aerobic workout or work a muscle group. That means its easy to try new exercises and equipment when its time to freshen up your workout routine. And the more choices you have, the easier it is to stick with your exercise program.

> **If you want to give your mind a rest, put your body to work.**

• **Relaxation.** If you want to give your mind a rest, put your body to work. Many of my patients report that time spent at the gym is deeply relaxing. Their focus is on simple physical tasks, such as lifting weights and breathing properly. Workouts are an oasis in a day of obligations.

Is joining a health club expensive? Only if you don't use your membership. To make sure you choose a club that's right for you, consider the following before signing a membership agreement:

Location. Join a club that's convenient to home or work. It's too easy to avoid working out if your club is too far out of your way.

Hours. Will you be able to work out at a time that's convenient for you? Can you take advantage of less crowded off-peak times?

Cleanliness. Check out the bathrooms and showers. Remember, it's supposed to be a *health* club. That means the facilities are cleaned regularly. Better clubs clean their changing, shower and restroom facilities throughout the day.

Staff. Do the people behind the reception counter greet you with a smile? Do they make eye contact? Or are they too busy comparing tans and muscle mass to notice you? You want to feel comfortable asking these people for help. After all, you'll be paying for it.

Atmosphere. Does everyone in the club look like a professional bodybuilder? Are there men and women working out? What kind of music is playing and how loud? Does the staff make an effort to "walk the floor" to answer questions or offer training tips? Each club has a distinct "personality." In this way, joining a health club is a little like having a roommate. Either you get along great, you put up with each other or you move out.

Stretching Area. Is there a separate area to stretch before your workout?

Weight Room. Are there enough free weights and weight machines to go around? What about cardiovascular equipment such as stairclimbers, treadmills, stationary bikes, rowing and skiing and elliptical motion machines? Is the equipment clean and in good repair? You want to be able to spend your time working out, not waiting in line.

Aerobics. Does the club offer aerobics classes? If so, ask for a class schedule. If you plan on being the Sultan of Step or the Queen of Kickboxing, make sure the only class isn't offered at 5 a.m. Also, ask about the aerobics instructor's certification. Look for credentials from the American Council on Exercise, the Aerobic Fitness Association of America or the Exercise Safety Council.

Extras:

Sports Leagues. Many clubs organize basketball, volleyball and racquetball leagues.

Swimming Pools. Check chlorination levels and cleaning schedules. Are swimming and water aerobics courses offered? How many lap lanes are available throughout the day and during lessons?

Childcare Services. More and more clubs are offering onsite childcare for parents who need someone to watch their kids while they work out. Many clubs contract with experienced daycare companies to maintain and staff the club's childcare facilities. Even so, make sure you check the childcare facility and staff with the same scrutiny you'd apply to a full-time daycare center. At a minimum, the staff must be certified for infant and child CPR training. Ask about fire, emergency and security procedures. Are staff required to have background checks? How often are toys and equipment cleaned? Ask about the sickness policy. Get the answers you need to have the peace of mind that your children will be safe and happy while you're taking some time for your own health and happiness.

Orientation Tours. Some clubs offer free orientation tours to show new members how to use the equipment. Make sure the advice comes from a certified personal trainer — not the receptionist.

Personal Training Programs. Many clubs offer one-on-one sessions with a personal trainer as an additional service. Working with a personal trainer is a great way to stay motivated and focused during your workout. Most clubs offer a complimentary training session and fitness evaluation to entice you to sign up for a series of personal training sessions. Others also throw in nutritional supplements and high-energy bars. But those incentives won't matter if you don't choose the right personal trainer for you. And that leads us to…

How to Choose a Personal Trainer

You want a trainer who listens to understand your needs and who takes the time to explain information in a way that you can understand.

Health clubs are overflowing with free advice from well-meaning members. The problem is that much of it is misguided or just plain wrong. It can also be dangerous. Push yourself too hard on a treadmill, lift too much weight or use bad form and you're bound to hurt yourself.

Learning how to exercise safely and efficiently is a good reason for working with a personal trainer. Hiring a personal trainer also makes sense if:

- You want to stay motivated and focused.
- You want a fitness routine customized to help you reach your health goals.

These days, a lot of people are calling themselves personal trainers. The hard part is choosing a personal trainer who's right for you. Here are some tips and criteria to keep in mind...

- **Credentials.** There was a time when all you needed to call yourself a personal trainer was a good body and a business card. Today, professional personal trainers are certified by nationally recognized fitness organizations. Look for credentials from the International Sports Science Association (ISSA), the American College of Sports Medicine (ACSM), the American Council on Exercise (ACE), the Institute for Aerobics Research or the National Strength and Conditioning Association.

- **Educational Background.** Want to work with a trainer who is committed to their profession? One indication is a bachelor's degree in health or exercise sciences. You also want someone who keeps up-to-date on fitness training and health information. Ask prospective trainers if they subscribe to any professional journals or attend continuing education classes or seminars.

- **CPR/First Aid Training.** If something goes wrong during your workout, can your trainer do more for you than dial 911?

- **Personality.** You are hiring a personal trainer to give you the motivation and information you need to benefit from a fitness routine. Being positive and enthusiastic is part of a personal trainer's job description. What matters is just how that enthusiasm is expressed through a trainer's personality. There's a huge difference between non-stop bubbly and non-stop intensity. You'll be paying this person to spend a lot of time with you, so make sure you have a good rapport.

- **Communication Skills.** An effective personal trainer needs superb communication skills. You want a trainer who listens to your needs and who takes the time to explain information in a way that you can understand. A trainer with a Ph.D. in exercise science is useless if they can't communicate their knowledge in a way that makes sense to you. There is no such thing as a stupid question. If a trainer makes you feel otherwise, find another trainer.

- **Gender.** Training is an up close and personal activity. Working with a trainer of the same or opposite sex may make a difference to you.

- **Fees.** Expect to pay between $50 and $100 an hour for a personal trainer. Ask about reduced rates for multiple sessions. What is the trainer's cancellation policy? How and when are you billed?

- **Availability.** Can the trainer accommodate your schedule? If you're not a morning person, don't expect yourself to get up at 5:30 a.m. to sweat with Sven.

5 Mental Health: Helpful Hints for Happiness

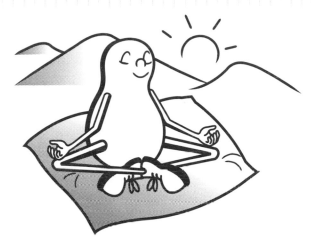

One of the principles of the Total Health program is that your mental health is just as important as your physical health. Here are some tips on how to preserve your emotional and social well-being and the importance of intellectual and spiritual growth.

Emotional and Social Well-Being

Seek and nurture healthy relationships. Choose your friends carefully. Look for people who value honesty and integrity. Look for people who build you up — not bring you down. Life is hard enough without inviting unhealthy, energy-draining personal and business relationships into your life.

Suppose you are a recovering alcoholic. In the past, you'd get drunk with the same group of friends on a regular basis. Now that you're trying to stay sober, you probably don't want to surround yourself with people who prefer to hang out in bars. And as much as you may like your old drinking buddies, the smarter choice is to cultivate friendships with people who understand your addiction and who support your decision not to drink.

Your life is directed by the choices you make. It isn't always easy to make the right choice. The important thing is to realize that you do have choices!

When it comes to business relationships, it doesn't matter whether you are a doctor, a mechanic or a roofing contractor. Eventually, we all face situations that raise moral and ethical dilemmas. Your life is directed by the choices you make. It isn't always easy to make the right choice. The important thing is to realize that you do have choices!

Intellectual Development

Commit to a lifetime of learning — professionally and personally. Want financial success? Provide increasingly better service to your customers or clients. Keep up with your profession's or trade's new trends, techniques and equipment. Attend continuing education seminars. Read professional journals and books. It doesn't matter whether you treat patients or repair cars. Strive to become the best at what you do. Your investment will pay off in higher self-esteem, confidence, job satisfaction and income.

Balance professional development with personal growth. Stimulate your brain with hobbies and activities that spark creativity. Write, draw, paint, play music, play chess, dance, sing. Too busy? Give your creative time the same respect you give your professional time. Pull out your day planner and set aside time for fun!

Bonus: Spend quality time with the most important people in your life by involving your spouse, significant other or children in your creative endeavors. You never know when you might spark a shared interest. That's what happened to me when my uncle came to visit. He was an artist and he always brought sketch pads and pencils for me and my siblings. Then he'd teach us how to draw. When I was four years old, he taught me how to play chess. I don't draw like Rembrandt or play chess like Kasparov, but that's not the point. Thanks to my uncle's gift of time, I discovered two creative outlets that I enjoy to this day.

Spiritual Growth

Contemplate your life's purpose. What are you here for? When you aren't clear about your life's purpose, you're likely to pass through life without direction. This lack of focus often leads to poor personal and business decisions, poor career choices, relationship problems, depression, eating disorders, substance abuse and a host of other life-draining distractions.

Set aside time on a daily basis to reflect on your purpose, dreams and goals in life.

When you are clear about your life's purpose, you can focus your energy towards achieving meaningful goals and dreams. Figuring out your purpose in life takes time and determination. Consider the following suggestions to help you get started...

Make time for self-renewal. Set aside time on a daily basis to reflect on your purpose, dreams and goals in life. If you believe in God or a higher power, you can pray for direction on how you can best use your talents to fulfill your purpose in life. It doesn't matter where you are — at home, commuting to work, on the golf course, in the shower — you can always take a few minutes to reflect on who you are, what you have accomplished in life and how you fit into the big picture.

Tip: Spend your self-renewal time focusing on love and goodness. Don't you spend enough time thinking about how much you have to do and how little time you have to do it? Isn't it demoralizing to watch the anger, injustice and violence on the nightly news? You cannot control the actions of others. But you can control your own thoughts and actions. Choose to dwell on what's right and good for a few minutes each day. It's good for the soul.

Love and serve others. This is one of the best ways to begin to discover your life's purpose. Regardless of your economic background, age, race or religion, you can love and serve others by showing concern and giving your time to people who are less fortunate.

Most of us won't live up to the good deeds of Mother Theresa, but we can experience the same joy and goodness just by serving the people closest to us. Nowhere is this principle's power more evident than in it's ability to shape the lives of children.

How do we describe a parent's job? A parent *raises* or *brings up* a child. Think about that for a moment. The job description calls for parents *to raise* children, *to bring them up*. Not tear them down. One of the easiest ways "to bring a child up" is to praise them for the things they do right!

You don't have to be a parent to make a tremendous impact on a child's life. Do you know any single mothers or fathers who are struggling to raise children? Simple gestures, such as including their kid in your own family function, can make all the difference.

I know because it happened to me. My dad left my mom when I was seven. I had two older brothers and a younger sister. My mom had spent 15 years as a housewife. She had no marketable skills — and now she had to support us. She went to work for minimum wage. There was no money for child care.

Fortunately, our neighbors across the street were concerned about our sudden change in fortune. They went out of their way to keep a close eye on me and my siblings while mom was at work. And they included us in many of their family activities. I remember going water-skiing and snow-mobiling. My neighbors even took me on their summer vacations.

It meant — and still means — the world to me that they opened their family to me. Over the years, I've come to realize that in many ways, they saved my life. Without a father and a mom who worked all the time, I needed the security of knowing that someone cared. God knows what kind of choices I would have made in life if I didn't have that security and love to fall back on.

Maybe my late grandmother's simple advice sums it up best. She said, "Every time I get depressed or start to feel sorry for myself, I just do something nice for someone else. It makes me feel a lot better." Thank you, Grandma Markham!

Serve your community. Community service is another great way to love and serve others. If you have kids in school, get involved and help support programs that improve the quality of education. Help with after-school programs that offer kids positive activities that keep them out of trouble.

Community-based organizations such as the YMCA, Boy Scouts, Girl Scouts and teen centers help kids develop leadership and teamwork skills. They also promote healthy ideas about the value of service to others. Business and civic organizations such as Rotary International, Kiwanis, Optimists, Lions Clubs and American Legion also give back to the community by raising money for a wide range of community service organizations.

One More Thing. . .

All of us come from different backgrounds and different life experiences. These experiences can fill our lives with light and joy — and they can trap us in unhealthy and sometimes dangerous behaviors.

If you suffer from behaviors or addictions that are keeping you from realizing your life's potential, you owe it to yourself and your loved ones to seek some professional help. If money is an issue, there are many city, county, state and federally funded programs that can help. There are also many 12-step support programs, such as Alcoholics Anonymous and Adult Children of Alcoholics, that meet on a regular basis.

6 Total Health Success Stories

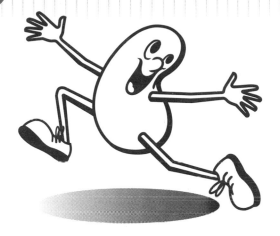

The Total Health program works for everyday people, every day. If you're looking for inspiration and motivation, you'll find it in the following pages...

I Can't Believe I Waited So Long

Sandy A.
Teacher
Age 60

I'm one of those people who's tried all the weight loss programs. I'd go on Slim Fast for two weeks and eat nothing else and gain weight. I tried the Diet Center, but it was too restrictive. And for two years, I kept losing and gaining anywhere from 30 to 50 pounds on Jenny Craig.

The problem with a lot of these expensive weight loss programs is that you don't start with regular food. It's all packaged stuff. And all you think about is eating regular food again. I was scared to death of eating regular food, because I knew I'd be back to my old ways. And that's what happened.

The Total Health program has done a lot to reduce my stress and increase my energy.

Total Health is the first program I've been on when I'm not always thinking about how long until I can get off of it. That's because this really isn't a diet. It's just the way you eat. After a while, it becomes second nature.

When I'm invited to dinner, I don't have to worry about the restaurant or that there is nothing on the menu I can eat. You just choose some meat, some vegetables or a salad and forget about the rest. It's that simple!

The Total Health program has also done a lot to reduce my stress and increase my energy. I used to come home from teaching totally stressed and I'd forage for anything. I was hungry for anything. Stale crackers, it didn't matter. Whatever it was, I'd shove it in my mouth.

Now, I come home and have a cheese stick and water. Before I'd come home and zone out in front of the television. Now at the end of the day, I have something left for my family. I feel really good now. We take walks every night.

I began working with Dr. Markham in November 1997. I started losing weight over Thanksgiving and Christmas and kept going. More than two years later, I've kept off 26 pounds. My husband is following the Total Health program, too. He's also lost weight and his cardiologist has been astonished at the way his cholesterol dropped from 230 to 170.

The hardest part of the Total Health program was making that first appointment with Dr. Markham. Now I can't believe I waited so long to pick up the phone.

A Second Chance at Life

Brad H.
Age 49
Computer Specialist

I have two birthdays. The first was April 7, 1950. My second was August 16, 1985. That's the day I had my heart attack. I was 35 at the time.

It was your classic heart attack. I was having dinner with my wife and a friend when the pain started in my left fingers and spread up my arm into my chest, which tightened like a vise. On the way to the hospital, I basically died in the back of the car. I was clinically dead until they revived me with those electronic paddles. People always ask how long I was gone. The only answer is 'long enough.'

When I regained consciousness, a cardiologist was standing over me with a clipboard. He started running down a checklist of lifestyle factors that cause heart attacks. The first question was 'How much alcohol do you drink?' I told him I didn't drink at all. Then, 'How much do you smoke?' I don't smoke. 'What about drugs?' I don't do drugs and never have. Period.

The doctor looked up from his clipboard. I was not making this easy. He wanted to understand why he was asking these questions of a 35 year old man who didn't drink, smoke or do drugs and who had no family history of heart problems. Finally he just said, 'Then, why the hell are you here?'

Good question. What did cause my heart attack?

In a word, "stress." In 1985, I was trying to move up the corporate ladder. Unfortunately, I was selling IBM typewriters in a world that was moving into computers. The fact that I weighed 240 pounds didn't help either. I knew I was about 30 pounds overweight, but I had always been a little on the heavy side. Besides, I was very active. Before my heart attack, I was actually running long distance, so I thought I was in really great shape.

There's nothing like death to give you a new perspective on life. You also get a lot of time to think while you watch your vital signs on the monitors next to your hospital bed. The way I saw it, I was getting a second chance at life. I had to lose the stress and the weight. It was a matter of survival.

Lowering my stress was the easy part. I quit my job while I was still in the hospital. The moment I did, the monitor showed my blood pressure dropping by 20 points. At first, I thought that losing the weight would be just as easy.

My doctors said to eat low fat foods and exercise. There was no formal instruction. As far as losing weight was concerned, I was on my own. For the next 15 years, I tried anything I thought would work.

I started with the Atkins diet, then the Diet Center and then Atkins again. Next I tried cutting all the fat, only to gain even more. At one point, I even went on a diet of grapefruit, eggs and spinach. I lost 85 pounds. But it all came back.

I was a human yo-yo. I'd starve myself on a diet. Then when I did eat, I'd eat twice as much. And the more weight I lost, the more I'd gain. There was never a moment I didn't think about food. Until I met Dr. Markham.

Ever since the heart attack, I've monitored my blood pressure regularly. One day at work it was up to 240/125. Given my history and my weight, which once again was at pre-heart attack levels, I was off to the Emergency Room to get checked out. I was told that if I didn't do something to lower my blood pressure, another heart attack or a stroke was just around the corner.

My company's nurse knew that I had worked out at the health club three to five times a week for years and never lost any weight. I was eating high quality food in reasonable amounts, but there was no weight loss. We agreed there was a clear connection between the food I was eating and my body's response to it. That's when she recommended that I check out one of Dr. Markham's presentations. Right away, I knew I found someone as passionate about my health as I was.

. . . I don't even think of food anymore. In fact, there are times when I have to look at my watch to remind myself to eat.

I started the Total Health program in May, 1999. Since then, I've lost 30 pounds without any sort of exercise whatsoever. My triglyceride count, which measures the amount of fat in blood, went from above 189 to below 50. And my blood pressure went from 240/125 down to 117/76.

I think of Total Health as an eating lifestyle because it's so easy to follow. The first day I had a headache from sugar withdrawal. But it went away within 24 hours. And from that day to this, I have never craved sugar of any kind. As long as you eat your protein and carbohydrates in the right combinations and portions, you can't go wrong.

Since I've adopted the Total Health eating lifestyle, I've dropped three notches on my belt. My metabolism has picked up and my mental focus has increased significantly. Best of all, I don't even think of food anymore. In fact, there are times when I have to look at my watch to remind myself to eat.

A New Way of Eating

Ellen M.
Physical Education Teacher
Age 50

In my profession, you are swamped with information about nutrition and exercise. It doesn't take long before you realize that no two experts really agree. So you have to go with what works for you, as long as it does no harm.

As a physical education teacher, I've always exercised daily, at least five and usually six days a week. Still, I'd always struggled to keep off an extra 10 to 20 pounds. Because I was getting plenty of exercise, I knew the key had to be what I was eating. So over the years I experimented with all sorts of diets. Most of them were different variations of the classic high carb diet, the stuff you'd always read in health and fitness magazines.

But following conventional wisdom didn't work. Losing weight on high carb diets was a struggle. In fact, I had to dramatically increase my level of exercise to keep from gaining!

I've seen a lot of fad diets come and go, so I was incredibly skeptical when friends invited me to one of Dr. Markham's free dinner lectures. I had already cut out bread and pasta for two weeks after glancing through *The Zone*. But that didn't do much for me, either.

I went to Dr. Markham's presentation out of pure curiosity. At the time I wanted to lose ten pounds. I wasn't planning on starting another program, but Total Health seemed so easy and straightforward that I had to give it a shot.

dropped 30 pounds and nearly two years later, I've kept it off.

One of the things I liked about Total Health is the clear menu choices. I also like being able to eat things that are not on any other diet. I still can't believe that I can eat open-faced double cheeseburgers. The first week, I had one every other night and lost three pounds!

After I dropped my ten pounds, I decided to go for ten more. And then another ten. I'd lost 30 pounds, but I was still cautious. In any diet, you can lose weight right away. My trouble was that I always gained it back. That hasn't been the case with Total Health. I dropped 30 pounds and nearly two years later, I've kept it off.

The difference I've discovered with Total Health is that it isn't a diet. It's a new way of eating. From time to time I've indulged myself with higher carb foods, but I've always been able to get back on track just by following the program. It's as easy as eating my next meal.

At first, it's hard for people to understand that following the Total Health eating program really works. The medical and nutritional community are locked into the notion that the traditional food pyramid still works. But that's changing.

My physician didn't like what I was doing, at first. But when my cholesterol dropped from 187 to 120, even he was impressed. He asked me what I was eating. I told him I was eating a lot of cheese. He said, 'then you didn't eat much meat, did you?' I said, as a matter of fact, I did. He said, 'whatever you're doing, keep it up, because it's working.'

A Balanced and Sensible Approach to Weight Loss

Troy M.
Manufacturing Manager
Age 54

I had been on high blood pressure medicine for two years when my wife, my daughter and I began consulting with Dr. Markham.

Both my wife and I had read *The Zone*. But that book was too technical. Dr. Markham's Total Health program was easy to learn. We also liked that it takes a balanced and sensible approach to weight loss. You don't feel that you're cheating if you don't measure out everything you put in your mouth. And if you do drift from the program, you can get back on track quickly.

This is not a diet where you drop 10 pounds and then go back to your old routine again. It's a new way of eating. It's a lifestyle change. And the more closely you follow the program, the faster your new eating routine will become second nature.

Starting a moderate exercise program also gives you an edge. You can lose weight just by following the eating program, but if you exercise, you'll reap the full benefits of what Total Health can do for you.

After I lost my first 30 pounds, my M.D. took me off my high blood pressure medication.

Another key to our success was that we made a commitment to learn the program and set up a plan. The first thing we did is purge the kitchen of all the foods we didn't need to eat. If you don't have the stuff in the house, you aren't even tempted to stray.

Then we planned out what we were going to eat each week. We created our own custom menus from the food list using chicken, meat and fish and the favorable carbs that we liked. We ate the same foods, but in different amounts because each of us had different protein and carbohydrate requirements.

After I lost my first 30 pounds, my M.D. took me off my high blood pressure medication. I went on to lose a total of 60 pounds and I've kept it off now for 16 months. My energy level has improved significantly. I don't need as much sleep as I used to and I'm not groggy in the morning anymore.

My wife has lost about 50 pounds and my daughter has dropped 25. She's a freshmen in high school and this program has helped boost her self-confidence. As her father,

I'm happy she can start benefiting from good eating habits earlier in life. Total Health is a nutritional foundation that she can build on.

My Husband Says I Saved His Life

Jackie P.
Contract Manager
Age 53

It's hard to believe that you can go through so much of your life with the wrong information. I've tried losing weight most of my life and all these years I was eating the wrong stuff.

> **People at work have told me how much more healthy I look. My skin looks better. I've also updated my wardrobe to go with my new body.**

I didn't think it was possible to lose weight and feel good at the same time. Every diet left me feeling exhausted and lousy. Some of them helped me lose weight, but only while I bought their prepackaged diet meals. As soon as I went back to the real food world, it was a constant struggle not to regain the weight.

This program is different. For starters, I have a lot more energy and I feel great! Total Health teaches you how to change your eating habits. It's not a diet, it's a way of eating, and you learn as you lose by eating the right kind of foods in the proper amounts. Everything you eat on this program, you buy at the supermarket.

Total Health is very easy to follow. And I like having a coach who can answer questions and show me how to make the program work for me.

I've followed Dr. Markham's program for six months and lost 42 pounds. People at work have told me how much more healthy I look. My skin looks better. I've also updated my wardrobe to go with my new body.

My husband is on the Total Health program, too. He was seeing an M.D. every three weeks to treat his high cholesterol and blood pressure. His doctor prescribed medication and a low – almost no – fat diet loaded with pasta. He lost a little weight but his blood pressure and cholesterol didn't budge.

Then he started following the Total Health program. Within three weeks, he went to his regular checkup. His doctor was astounded that his blood pressure and cholesterol levels were all down to normal. To date, my husband has lost 60 pounds. He's off his blood pressure medication and only sees his M.D. every six months for monitoring.

My husband tells me that I literally saved his life. And he looks great! I've been married 30 years and it's like I have a new husband.

I Lost 21 Pounds in Four Weeks on Fast Food!

Bob P.
Insurance Broker
Age: 47

In September 1997, I discovered that serious blood pressure problems were going to delay some minor surgery that I needed. Reluctantly, I started taking blood pressure medication and for three months it brought my blood pressure under control.

Then it stopped working. My blood pressure spiked and I got so frustrated that I threw the pills out. I've always hated taking medications and to get me on blood pressure medication in the first place was like pulling teeth.

On a good day, my blood pressure was up to 157/105. Not horrible, but not good. I was about to go back to my doctor for a new prescription, when a good deed led me to Dr. Markham's Total Health program.

My mother had attended one of Dr. Markham's presentations and I'd agreed to take her for a free consultation. As a favor to my mother, Dr. Markham gave me a customized menu, too. No obligation.

I never expected this program to work. I'd been trying to lose the same 25 pounds for about five years. I've tried no-fat and low-fat diets. I've listened to all sorts of well-meaning, but ultimately bad advice about losing weight. And when I did lose weight, it always came back within a couple weeks.

Since I started the Total Health program, I've completely revised my expectations of myself upwards. My weight dropped from 255 to 200 pounds. My blood pressure is down. My waist size is now 36. And I have the confidence and energy to start a regular exercise program.

So when I began dropping weight on Dr. Markham's Total Health program, I was floored! For one thing, the program seemed too easy. For another, I'd never lost more than two pounds in one week — no matter what I did. All I did was follow my menu options and *I lost seven pounds my first week!* By week four, I'd lost 21 pounds. My waist sized dropped from 42 to 38.

Then one night I took my blood pressure. It was 125/82. I've been off blood pressure medication ever since.

The Total Health program is unlike anything I've tried before. I eat something every three hours, so I never feel hunger pangs. And I check in with Dr. Markham once a week to help me stay on track.

What I like most about the Total Health program is that it works in the real world. I work at a ferocious pace and

I'm never home. The way my schedule is, I'm almost always using the fast food options. That's the part most people just can't believe: I lost 21 pounds in four weeks on fast food.

Since I started the Total Health program, I've completely revised my expectations of myself upwards. My weight dropped from 255 to 200 pounds. My blood pressure is down. My waist size is now 36. And I now have the confidence and energy to start a regular exercise program. For a 47-year old guy who moves around as much as I do, I think that's pretty damn good.

Appendix I: Commit to Health and Happiness!

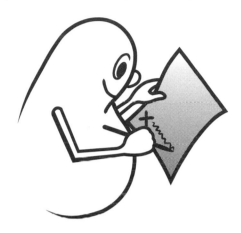

Here's one contract you won't have to run by an attorney. It's your own personal contract for health and happiness. Make a copy of this contract, sign it, and read it daily. Use it to reaffirm your desire and commitment to live in Total Health and renew your pledge to participate in life to the best of your abilities.

Remember, it's your absolute right to be healthy and happy! It's my deepest wish that this book and the Total Health program helps you take the first step towards lifelong health and happiness.

Total Health
Contract for Health & Happiness

I, _____, hereby declare that I promise myself and my loved ones to nourish my body with a proper diet, and to enjoy the lifelong benefits of physical and mental health through exercise, intellectual development and spiritual growth.

This commitment will help me maintain and enjoy the quality of life that I most certainly deserve for participating in life to the best of my abilities.

Signed:_____ Date:_____

Appendix II: Total Health Before and After Photos

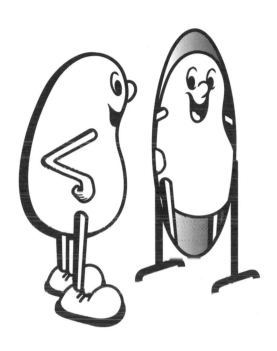

Lost 56 Pounds in 6 Months

BEFORE

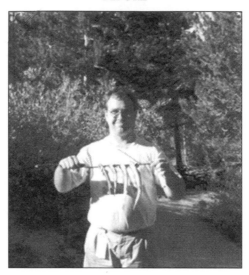

AFTER

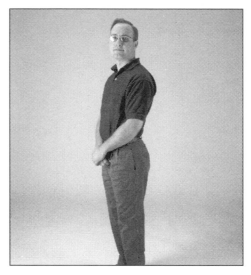

Steve L.
Publishing Executive
Age 34

Lost 72 Pounds in 8 Months

BEFORE

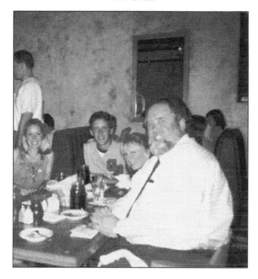

AFTER

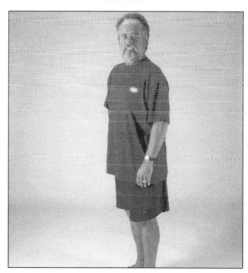

Greg B.
Insurance Agent
Age 49

Lost 50 Pounds in 4 Months

BEFORE

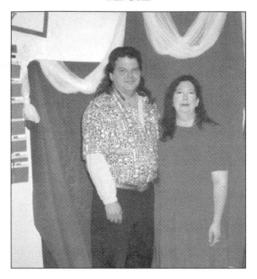

AFTER

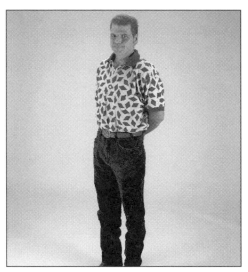

Jerry K.
Retail Sales
Age 41

Lost 75 Pounds in 15 Months

BEFORE

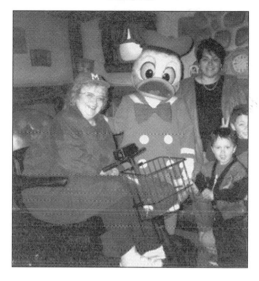

AFTER

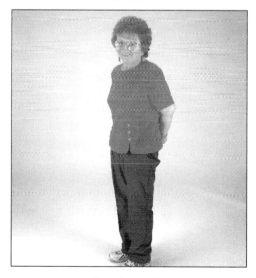

Barabara S.
Retired
Age 53

Lost 24 Pounds in 6 Months

BEFORE

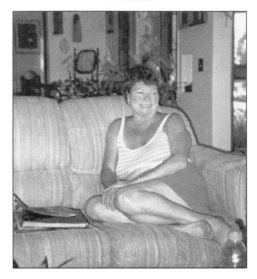

AFTER

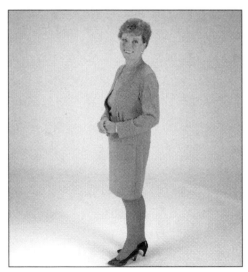

Judy A.
Account Executive
Age 60

Lost 52 Pounds in 7 Months

BEFORE

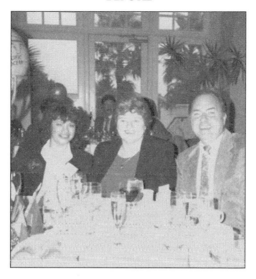

AFTER

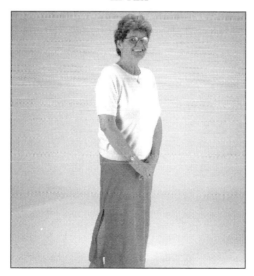

Sue M.
Accounting Clerk
Age 59

Lost 57 Pounds in 5 Months

BEFORE

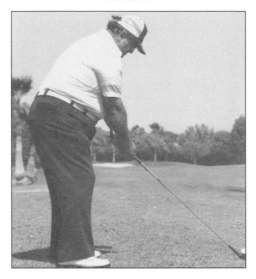

AFTER

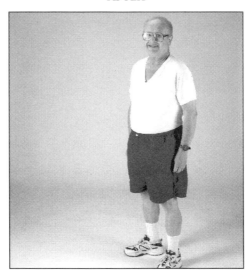

George P.
Retired
Age 69

Bibliography

Anderson, Bob. *Stretching.* Bolinas: Shelter Publications, 1984.

Audette, Ray with Troy Gilchrist. *Neanderthin: Eat Like a Caveman to Achieve a Lean, Strong, Healthy Body.* New York: St. Martins Press, 1999.

Brzycki, Matt. *Maximize Your Training: Insights from Leading Strength and Fitness Professionals.* Chicago: Masters Press, 2000.

D'Adamo, Peter with Catherine Whitney. *Eat Right for Your Type: The Individualized Diet Solution to Staying Healthy, Living Longer & Achieving Your Ideal Weight.* New York: G.P. Putnam, 1996.

Daoust, Joyce and Gene Daoust. *40-30-30 Fat Burning Nutrition: The Dietary Hormonal Connection to Permanent Weight Loss and Better Health.* Del Mar, California: Wharton Publishing, 1996.

Dufty, William. *Sugar Blues.* New York: Warner Books, 1976.

Eades, Michael and Mary Eades. *Protein Power.* New York: Bantam Books, 1996.

Erasmus, Udo. *Fats and Oils: The Complete Guide to Fats and Oils in Health and Nutrition.* Vancouver: Alive Books, 1986.

Gittleman, Ann. *The 40-30-30 Phenomenon: The Easy-to-Follow Diet Plan Tailored for Individual Needs.* New Canaan, Connecticut: Keats Publishing, 1997.

Guyton, Arthur. *Textbook of Medical Physiology, 7th ed.* Philadelphia: W.B. Saunders, 1986.

Haas, Robert. *Eat to Win: The Sports Nutrition Bible.* New York: Rawson Associates, 1983.

Hecker, Arthur ed. *Clinics in Sports Medicine: Nutritional Aspects of Exercise.* Philadelphia: W.B. Saunders Company, 1984.

Heller, Richard and Rachael Heller. *The Carbohydrate Addict's Diet : The Lifelong Solution to Yo-Yo Dieting.* New York: Penguin, 1991.

Heller, Richard and Rachael Heller. *Carbohydrate-Addicted Kids : Help Your Child or Teen Break Free of Junk Food and Sugar Cravings — for Life!* New York: HarperCollins, 1997.

Neporent, Liz and Suzanne Schlosberg. *Weight Training for Dummies.* New York: IDG Books Worldwide, 1997.

Sears, Barry with Bill Lawren. *The Zone: A Dietary Road Map to Lose Weight Permanently, Reset Your Genetic Code, Prevent Disease, Achieve Maximum Physical Performance, Enhance Mental Productivity.* New York: ReganBooks, 1995.

Sizer, Frances, and Eleanor Whitney. *Nutrition: Concepts and Controversies, 6th ed.* St. Paul: West Publishing Company, 1994.

Weil, Andrew. *Natural Health, Natural Medicine: A Comprehensive Manual for Wellness and Self-Care.* New York: Houghton Mifflin, 1995.

Weil, Andrew. *Eating Well for Optimum Health: The Essential Guide to Food, Diet, and Nutrition.* New York: Alfred A. Knopf, 2000.

Vigilante, Kevin and Mary Flynn. *Low-Fat Lies : High Fat Frauds & the Healthiest Diet in the World.* Washington: Lifeline Press, 1999.

Zarins, Bertram, ed. *Clinics in Sports Medicine: Olympic Sports Medicine.* Philadelphia: W.B. Saunders Company, 1983.

Index

A

Addiction of food, 21
Adult Children of Alcoholics, 83
Aerobic exercise, 64–66
Aerobic Fitness Association of
    America, 73
Airway dilation, 31
Alcoholics Anonymous, 83
Alpha linoleic acid (ALA), 34
American Council on Exercise
    (ACE), 73
American Society of Clinical
    Nutrition, 12
Amputation, 24
Anemia, 47
Antioxidants, 49 50
Arachidonic acid (AA), 34

B

Biochemical reactions, 21–24
Blackburn, George, 12
Blindness, 24
Blood clotting, 31
Blood sugar regulation
    eating intervals and, 36–37
    increase of energy through, 15
Body mass, 35–36
Bread/pasta, 59
Breast cancer, 12
Broccoli extract, 51
Butter, 33

C

Caffeine, 53
Calcium, 47, 51
Cancer
    fiber intake and, 58–59
    obesity and, 12

Canola oil, 34
Carbohydrates
    contribution to obesity by, 26–30
    daily grams needed, 36–37
    exercise and, 63–65
    fiber-rich fruits/vegetables, 59
    high-/low-glycemic, 29
    as macronutrients, 26
Case studies, 85–99, 105–112
Cell growth, 31
Cellulose, 57–58
Chiropractic, 68
Cholesterol
    fiber intake and, 58
    testimonials regarding, 93
    Total Health diet and, 39–42
Coffee, 53
Colon cancer
    fiber intake and, 58–59
    obesity and, 12
Community organizations, 82–83
Contract for health/happiness, 102
Costs
    federally funded programs, 83
    of personal trainers, 76
    of supplements, 42
    of weight loss industry, 13
Council for Responsible Nutrition, 42

D

Death, 12
Dehydration, 53–54
Delta 5 desaturase enzyme, 32
Delta 6 desaturase enzyme, 32, 34
Depression, 79–80
Diabetes
    excess insulin and, 23–24
    obesity and, 12
Dietary Reference Intakes (DRIs), 47

Dietary Supplement Health and Education Act of 1994, 43

E

Eades, Mary, 15
Eades, Michael, 15
Eating disorders, 79–80
Eating intervals, 36–37
Eggs, 34, 38
Eicosanoids
    avoidance of alpha linoleic acid (ALA), 34
    balance of good/bad, 30–32
    eicosapentaenoic acid (EPA), 35
    monitoring of arachidonic acid(AA), 34
Eicosapentaenoic acid (EPA), 35
Endurance, 31
Energy
    ginseng and, 52
    increase through blood sugar regulation, 14–15
    testimonials regarding, 86
Enter the Zone, 15
Enzymes, 32, 34
Exercise
    aerobic, 65–66
    benefits of, 62–64
    choosing health clubs, 70–74
    choosing personal trainers, 74–76
    passive, 68–69
    resistance, 66–67
    U.S. Surgeon General's report on, 61
Exercise Safety Council, 73

F

Fats
    cholesterol and, 39
    as macronutrients, 26
    and production of eicosanoids, 30

Fatty acids
    avoidance of alpha linoleic acid (ALA), 34
    eicosapentaenoic acid (EPA), 35
    linoleic acid, 33–34
    trans, 33–34
Fiber, 57–60
Fish oil, 34
Flaxseed oil, 34
Folic acid, 47
Food
    composition of, 25
    as a drug, 21–24
Food and Nutrition Board of the Institute of Medicine, 46
Free radicals, 49–50

G

Ginkgo biloba, 52
Ginseng, 52
Glucagon
    aerobic exercise and, 64–65
    eating of proteins and, 28–29
    release/effect of, 22–24
Glucose, 26–30
Grape seed extract, 51
Gum, 57

H

Happiness. See Mental health
Health clubs, 70–74
Heart disease
    due to diabetes, 24
    fiber intake and, 58
    HDLs and, 40–41
    testimonials regarding, 87–90
    trans fatty acids and, 33–34
Heart rate monitor, 65–66
Hemicellulose, 57–58
Hemorrhoids, 58

Herbs, 52
High blood pressure
    obesity and, 12
    testimonials regarding, 89–90, 94, 96–99
Hormones
    eicosanoids, 30–35
    Human growth hormone (HGH), 67
    release/effect of, 22–24
    response to food, 26–30
Human growth hormone (HGH), 67
Hypoglycemia, 28

I

Immune system, 31–32
Impotency, 24
Inflammation, 31
Institute for Aerobics Research, 75
Insulin
    activation of delta 5 desaturase by, 32
    aerobic exercise and, 64
    cholesterol and, 39
    fiber intake and, 58
    release/effect of, 22–24
    resistance to, 27–28
    water retention and, 56
Intellectual development, 78–79
International Sports Science
    Association (ISSA), 75
Iron supplements, 48

K

Kidney failure
    due to diabetes, 24
lack of water and, 53–54

L

Lignin, 57–58
Linoleic acid, 32–33

avoidance of alpha, 34
and delta 5 desaturase, 32
and production of eicosanoids, 30, 32
Lycopene, 51

M

Macronutrients, 25–26
Mental health
    contract for health/happiness, 102
    intellectual development, 78–79
    relationships and, 77–78
    spiritual growth, 79–83
Menu option samples, 38
Metabolic rate
    exercise and, 64, 66–67
    testimonials regarding, 90
Metamucil, 60
Micronutrients, 25
    choosing appropriate, 49–52
    minerals, 43–45
    overdoses of, 48
    popularity of, 42, 43
    supplied by Total Health diet, 47–48
    vitamins, 43–45
    water, 53–57
Minerals, 43–45
    chelated/trace minerals, 51
    choosing appropriate, 49–52
    deficiencies, 45–46

N

National Strength and
    Conditioning Association, 75

O

Obesity
    in America, 11–13
    exercise in America and, 61

glucagon as fat-burner, 28–29
as health risk factor, 12, 14
high-carbohydrates meals
and, 27–30
water intake and, 54
Oils. See Fatty acids
Olive oil, 34
Osteoporosis, 57
Oxygen flow
eicosanoids and, 31
exercise and, 65
ginkgo biloba and, 52

P

Pain, 31
Passive exercise, 68–69
Pasta, 59
Pectin, 57
Personal relationships/growth,
77–78
Personal trainers, 74–76
Phytonutrients, 50–51
Proanthocyanidins, 51
Protein Power, 15
Proteins
daily grams needed, 36–37
eicosanoid balance and, 32
as macronutrients, 26
requirements of, 35–36
stimulation of glucagon
release, 28–29, 32

R

Recommended Dietary
Allowances(RDAs), 46–47
Resistance exercise, 64, 66–67
Rexall's Bios Life, 60

S

Sears, Barry, 15
Sesame oil, 34
Soybean oil, 34
Spiritual growth, 79–83
Stretching exercise. See Passive exercise
Stroke, 12
Sulforaphane, 51
Supplements. See Micronutrients

T

Testimonials, 85–99, 105–112
Tomato extract, 51
Total Health Pack supplements 49,
52, 59
Trans fatty acids, 33–34
Triglycerides, 39–41

V

Vitamins, 43–45
antioxidants, 49–50
choosing appropriate, 49–52
deficiencies, 45
phytonutrients, 50–51

W

Water, 53–58, 60
Web site of Total Health, 19, 30, 38
Weight loss. See also Obesity
costs of, 13
importance of eating intervals, 36–37
regular exercise and, 62–67
sample protein/carbohydrate
requirements for, 37
testimonials, 85–99
Weight training. See Resistance exercise

About the Author

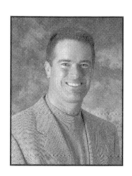 Dr. Douglas Markham is a 1984 graduate of the Palmer College of Chiropractic in Davenport, Iowa. A former chiropractor for the U.S. Rugby team and an All-American wrestler, Dr. Markham specializes in nutrition and musculo-skeletal disorders. His offices are located on the Los Robles Regional Medical Center Campus in Thousand Oaks, California.

Speeches and Corporate Wellness Programs

Dr. Markham's Total Health program is a balanced nutrition and exercise program that has helped hundreds of patients take control of their health. He lectures extensively on how to use everyday foods and exercise to achieve permanent weight loss, boost energy and improve longevity. To inquire about speaking engagements and corporate wellness programs, please call (800) 891-5165.

Start Living in Total Health Today!

Order your Total Health weight loss and wellness menus online at

www.totalhealthdoc.com

Dr. Markham's Total Health menus make it easy to unlock your body's natural ability to burn fat, boost your energy and stay healthy.

- All menus and food choices are customized for your body size, weight loss and health goals.

- Easy-to-follow food options for breakfast, lunch, dinner and snacks make it easy to know what to eat and when.

- An extensive list of everyday protein-rich, favorable-carbohydrate foods offer variety and flexibility.

- Food preparation tips for dining out in Total Health.

- Convenient "fast-food" options for drive-thru dining.

- Total Health success tips to speed your progress.

Hundreds of patients have used Dr. Markham's Total Health menus to eat their way to lower body fat and better health. Join them today! You'll be amazed at just how easy it is to live in Total Health.

To order your customized Total Health menu, visit

www.totalhealthdoc.com

Total Health Pack™
Dietary Supplements

Total Health Pack dietary supplements are custom-designed to enhance the effectiveness of Dr. Markham's Total Health program with an essential blend of vitamins, minerals, herbs and fiber.

A 30-day supply of Total Health Pack supplements includes both the Morning and Evening Formulas.

Total Health Pack Morning Formula is a powerful combination of essential vitamins, minerals, herbs and fiber formulated for peak daytime performance. Benefits include increased energy and metabolism, immune system support, enhanced brain function and antioxidant protection.

Total Health Pack Evening Formula delivers a select blend of vitamins, minerals, herbs and fiber to replenish vital micronutrients while you sleep. Benefits include more restful and rejuvenating sleep, increased immune system support and antioxidant protection.

To order Total Health Pack dietary supplements, use the order form in this book, call toll-free (800) 891-5165, or visit **www.totalhealthdoc.com**

Give the Gift of Total Health

Dr. Markham's Total Health program is a remarkably easy, effective and safe way to take control of your health and stay healthy.

It also makes a great gift!

Give a copy of *Total Health: How to Unlock Your Body's Natural Ability to Burn Fat, Stay Healthy & Boost Your Energy* to your friends and family.

To order gift copies of *Total Health,* use the order form in this book, call (800) 891-5165, or visit www.totalhealthdoc.com

TOTAL HEALTH 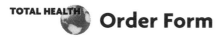 Order Form

Fax orders: (805) 480-0580. Fax this form.

Telephone orders: Call toll-free at 1-800-891-5165. Have your credit card ready.

Online orders: www.totalhealthdoc.com

Mail orders: Total Health Care Partners, Inc., 3835-R East
Thousand Oaks Blvd., Suite 130, Westlake Village, CA 91362-3637.

Please send more information on:

❑ Speeches and seminars

❑ Corporate weight loss and wellness consulting

❑ Total Health Pack™ Dietary Supplements

❑ Favorable-carbohydrate and protein-rich food products

❑ B.A.R. (Bungee-Aerobic-Resistance) Home Exercise Program

❑ Online weight loss and wellness program

❑ Total Health newsletter

❑ Health care practice consulting

Please send the following items:

Quantity	Item	Cost	Total
☐	*Total Health* Book	$19.95 / each	_____
☐	Total Health Pack™ (30 Day Supply)	$34.95 / each	_____
☐	B.A.R. (Bungee-Aerobic-Resistance) Home Exercise Program	$29.95 / each	_____
	Sales Tax	(CA residents 7.25%)	_____
	Shipping/Handling	$3 for first item; add $1.75 for each additional item	_____
		Total	_____

Payment Options (Select One)

Make checks payable to Total Health Care Partners, Inc.

❑ Check   ❑ Money Order   ❑ Visa   ❑ Master Card

Credit Card Number: _____ Exp. Date: _____

Card Holder Name: _____

Name: _____

Address:_____

City:_____ State: _____ Zip Code: _____

Phone: (   )_____(   )_____ Fax: _____
             Daytime   Evening

E-Mail Address: _____

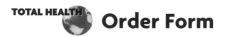

Order Form

TOTAL HEALTH

Fax orders: (805) 480-0580. Fax this form.

Telephone orders: Call toll-free at 1-800-891-5165. Have your credit card ready.

Online orders: www.totalhealthdoc.com

Mail orders: Total Health Care Partners, Inc., 3835-R East Thousand Oaks Blvd., Suite 130, Westlake Village, CA 91362-3637.

Please send more information on:

❑ Speeches and seminars

❑ Corporate weight loss and wellness consulting

❑ Total Health Pack™ Dietary Supplements

❑ Favorable-carbohydrate and protein-rich food products

❑ B.A.R. (Bungee-Aerobic-Resistance) Home Exercise Program

❑ Online weight loss and wellness program

❑ Total Health newsletter

❑ Health care practice consulting

Please send the following items:

Quantity	Item	Cost	Total
☐	*Total Health* Book	$19.95 / each	_____
☐	Total Health Pack™ (30 Day Supply)	$34.95 / each	_____
☐	B.A.R. (Bungee-Aerobic-Resistance) Home Exercise Program	$29.95 / each	_____
	Sales Tax	(CA residents 7.25%)	_____
	Shipping/Handling	$3 for first item; add $1.75 for each additional item	_____
		Total	_____

Payment Options (Select One)

Make checks payable to Total Health Care Partners, Inc.

❑ Check ❑ Money Order ❑ Visa ❑ Master Card

Credit Card Number: _____ Exp. Date: _____

Card Holder Name: _____

Name: _____

Address: _____

City: _____ State: _____ Zip Code: _____

Phone: ( )_____ ( )_____ Fax: _____
       Daytime   Evening

E-Mail Address: _____

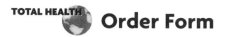

TOTAL HEALTH **Order Form**

Fax orders: (805) 480-0580. Fax this form.
Telephone orders: Call toll-free at 1-800-891-5165. Have your credit card ready.
Online orders: www.totalhealthdoc.com
Mail orders: Total Health Care Partners, Inc., 3835-R East
Thousand Oaks Blvd., Suite 130, Westlake Village, CA 91362-3637.

Please send more information on:

❑ Speeches and seminars
❑ Corporate weight loss and wellness consulting
❑ Total Health Pack™ Dietary Supplements
❑ Favorable-carbohydrate and protein-rich food products

❑ B.A.R. (Bungee-Aerobic-Resistance) Home Exercise Program
❑ Online weight loss and wellness program
❑ Total Health newsletter
❑ Health care practice consulting

Please send the following items:

Quantity	Item	Cost	Total
☐	*Total Health* Book	$19.95 / each	_____
☐	Total Health Pack™ (30 Day Supply)	$34.95 / each	_____
☐	B.A.R. (Bungee-Aerobic-Resistance) Home Exercise Program	$29.95 / each	_____
	Sales Tax	(CA residents 7.25%)	_____
	Shipping/Handling	$3 for first item; add $1.75 for each additional item	_____
		Total	_____

Payment Options (Select One)
Make checks payable to Total Health Care Partners, Inc.
❑ Check   ❑ Money Order   ❑ Visa   ❑ Master Card

Credit Card Number: _____ Exp. Date: _____

Card Holder Name: _____

Name: _____

Address: _____

City: _____ State: _____ Zip Code: _____

Phone: (   ) _____ (   ) _____ Fax: _____
Daytime   Evening
E-Mail Address: _____

Notes

Notes